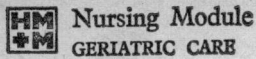 Nursing Module
GERIATRIC CARE

To all who grow old in Lambeth

SERIES EDITOR
Kathleen M. Berry, SRN SCM RNT AcDipEd

In the same series
Psychiatric Care
Obstetric Care
Community Care

Nursing Modules

Geriatric Care

Fiona McLeod, SRN HV Cert
Formerly Acting Ward Sister,
the South-Western Hospital, Geriatric
Department of St. Thomas's Hospital,
London, and Geriatric Liaison Health
Visitor, London Borough of Lambeth

HM + M Publishers
AYLESBURY, ENGLAND

© Fiona McLeod 1976

First edition, published by
H M + M Publishers Ltd,
Milton Road, Aylesbury, Buckinghamshire, England

ISBN 0 85602 026 5

Manufactured in Great Britain by
Hunt Barnard Printing Ltd,
Aylesbury, Buckinghamshire, England

Contents

Preface vii

1 Introducing Geriatrics 1
2 Growing Old 4
3 The Elderly Within the Community 14
4 The Diseases and Hazards of Old Age 23
5 The Geriatric Department 71
6 Old People as Patients 82
7 Aspects of Nursing Care 102
8 Rehabilitation 129
9 Return to the Community 153
10 Geriatric Care – The Present and the Future 172

Index 176

Preface

This book is one of four written with the object of providing guidance for student nurses undertaking the various options of experience required in their general training. These four options or modules of experience – geriatrics, obstetrics, psychiatry and community care – are not to be considered as separate entities but as complementary to one another and designed to provide an opportunity for student nurses to see their work in the broad human setting, including both the hospital and the community.

The aim of this book is to introduce the reader to the idea that geriatric care is more than the nursing of elderly people in a hospital ward. For the successful care of her patients the nurse must not only understand their medical condition but also their social background, expectations and special needs. The book builds up a picture of old people as members of the community, highlights the problems of old age and the admission of the elderly to hospital and outlines the specialised care that is available in hospital and the community. It is hoped that the nurse's experience in the Geriatric Department will not be limited to nursing in the wards but that she will have an opportunity to visit patients in their homes and to work in a day hospital.

Geriatric nursing is essentially the basic nursing taught in Schools of Nursing and it is without the drama and technicality of acute nursing care, which to some is its attraction. It gives the nurse an opportunity to develop her skills of patience, observation and ingenuity and allows her to work as part of a team with the doctors, physiotherapists, occupational therapists, health and social workers. This book will prepare the nurse for the experience of working with old people and suggestions for further reading are given at the end of each chapter for those readers who wish to study particular aspects of geriatric care in greater depth.

May 1976   FIONA MCLEOD

Acknowledgements

I would like to thank Jean Exton-Smith, Director of Nurse Education, Barnet Area Health Authority, for her advice and help in correcting the manuscript, Dr T. C. Picton Williams who advised on Chapter 4 and my husband, Michael, for his encouragement and patience while this book was being written. Susan Hales drew the illustrations.

1. Introducing Geriatrics

Until comparatively recently, elderly people who fell ill were often considered to be fit only for admission to hospital for 'chronic' care and were described as being senile; for some this unfortunate image of the elderly sick lingers on today. Lack of any positive treatment in the chronic wards reduced the patients to a state that justified the common image of their total incapacity and mental confusion. Over the last 20 to 30 years a completely new approach to the problems and possibilities of old age has developed. Careful assessment and diagnosis of illness and disability have shown that people admitted to geriatric wards can be treated, rehabilitated and can return to the community to live independently. The distinctive aim of geriatric care is to improve function so that the patient can live as normal a life as possible within any personal limitation.

Geriatrics is the term that is used for the medical and nursing care of elderly people. Gerontology is the scientific study of old age and the process of ageing. Rehabilitation and re-ablement are words commonly used in geriatric departments to describe the various processes used to restore confidence and function to the elderly patient and to prevent further disability. Whether a person qualifies for geriatric rather than general medical care depends more upon the nature of the condition than on the chronological age of the patient. Geriatric care attaches as much importance to the social condition of the patient as it does to the medical disorder, for it is of little value to make a person fit and mobile if her house is in such poor condition that within a week of her return home she falls and has to be re-admitted to hospital.

The very nature of geriatric medicine means that it cannot operate only within the confines of the hospital. Geriatric hospitals and day centres should be in the midst of the community they serve and not hidden away in the country, as are many of the older mental institutions, or aloof from the community as are some of the highly specialised units of the teaching hospitals. The community nursing and social services are as important a part of geriatric care as the hospital staff, for without their support many elderly people would be unable to continue living independently. These services also have an important preventive function in that they care for elderly people before they ever reach hospital. A recent development in this chain of care is the day hospital, where elderly people can receive the specialised care that only the hospital can provide while still living at home. In this way admission to hospital may be delayed or prevented, while relatives are relieved of much of the burden of support. The day hospital can also shorten the time that patients need for treatment as inpatients, while enabling their return to the community to be a more gradual process.

Geriatrics is a young and often misunderstood branch of medicine and its status within the medical profession is poor. This lack of prestige, which may be symptomatic of a society dominated by youth, shows itself in poorly equipped buildings often sited away from the main district hospitals. Recruitment of staff is difficult and this discourages those who are enthusiastic.

Within the community the elderly suffer because no one part of the National Health Service or the local authority Social Services Department is responsible for their needs as a group. A new-born baby, by law, must be visited by a health visitor during the earlier days of its life and from then on, throughout infancy and at school, each child is regularly examined by a doctor. This care is common for both healthy and sick children; for the socially deprived and the materially affluent. Adults are normally able to live independently without recourse to support from the social or health services, but the elderly, whose need for the services is often the greatest, have no adequate way, as yet, of being identified and helped. Some local authorities offer screening facilities for retired people but those who attend voluntarily are often not those in serious need. A small minority may come to the notice of the social services department through requests from general practitioners, neighbours, clergy or voluntary workers, but all the evidence suggests that there are many elderly people living in the community who would benefit from the services provided by the local authority and the voluntary agencies but do not ask for help through pride or ignorance of their entitlement.

This poor image of geriatric care may give the nurse a false impression of what nursing the elderly entails. Although there are still many hospitals with inadequate facilities, so much has been said and written recently about the care of the elderly that few hospitals can have resisted the changes brought about by this upsurge of interest. Geriatric nursing is no longer a continuous round of treating or preventing pressure sores and changing the incontinent patient. In geriatric wards the nurse has the chance to care for the acutely-ill patient, to assist with rehabilitation and to use her ingenuity to contribute towards an enlightened atmosphere in the long-stay wards. She will also learn to care for the dying and will come to appreciate the problems experienced by the relatives of elderly patients. Outside the ward, the nurse has a major part to play in running the day hospital and in caring for the elderly in the community. Geriatric care has come a long way in the last 30 years.

For further reading

Felstein, I. *Later life: Geriatrics Today and Tomorrow*. Penguin Books 1969

2. Growing Old

Geriatric care, like paediatric care, is concerned with the specialised needs of an age group rather than the care of patients with certain diseases. Just as it is essential to understand the normal development of the child when working in a children's ward so it is important to know something of the process of ageing, or senescence, when caring for elderly people in a geriatric ward not least because many elderly people and their relatives may assume too easily that disability is the result of ageing, while in fact it may result from a condition that can be treated.

One of the dangers of grouping elderly people together is to presume that they will age at the same rate and in a similar way. Ageing depends on genetic make-up (inherited factors) as well as the effect of circumstance and climate upon the individual during her lifetime. Some of the signs of apparent ageing may be due to disease, as, for example, in an elderly woman with thinning hair and dry pallid skin who may be suffering from hypothyroidism (myxoedema) rather than the effects of ageing on her hair follicles and complexion. It is important in geriatrics to consider a person to be of a certain biological age rather than of a chronological age, for ageing is not a continuous process. Some cells age faster than others; others, like red blood corpuscles, will continue to die and be replaced until the body dies, but some more highly complicated cells, such as those in the brain, die (or atrophy) and are not replaced. In normal circumstances the body is able to function quite adequately on half or less of the specialised cells that make up its different organs but in times of stress, such as during an illness, the reserves may be insufficient and the functioning of the organs will be impaired. The slow process of cell destruction is known as involution, which may be speeded up by disease, such as hypertension, or outside factors such as a working life spent in a dirty factory. Some people look old at 60 while others retain a comparatively youthful appearance at 80.

Physical changes

1 *General appearances*

As much as three inches in height may be lost with age, due partly to atrophy of the intervertebral discs which narrows the space between the vertebral bodies and partly because elderly people adopt a stooping posture, which itself may be a sign of muscle weakness. In some elderly people soft tissue continues to grow (hypertrophy), and can cause, for example, an unsightly bulbous nose and large ear lobes. The skin loses its elasticity and natural oiliness and hangs loosely over the bones. Great care must be taken when helping an elderly person to wash to ensure that skin folds are kept clean and dry. Elderly women may be worried by the reddish patches that look like bruising which appear beneath the skin, particularly on the forearms. These marks, called ecchymoses, are due to haemorrhages from the fragile blood capillaries under the skin, and are of no significance. Senile warts also occur on the skin. There is generally a thinning and loss of hair but the age at which these occur, as with greying, seems to depend largely on genetic factors. Elderly women may develop coarse facial hair, which if it is very unsightly can be removed with depilatory creams or by shaving. Loss of teeth and failure to wear dentures cause the skin over the jaws and gums to sink in, which can affect the speech.

2 *Bones, joints and muscles*

Bones become less dense and more brittle with age as the result of chemical changes. This is particularly significant because fractures of the long bones may occur with very little trauma.

Muscles become weaker and wasted with less use and movements are generally slower and more purposeful. Poor posture means that some muscles are badly used, and obese people, particularly, adopt a 'wide-based' waddling gait to overcome their unsteadiness which reduces their mobility further. The reflexes of elderly people are slower and fine movements less accurate, which may lead to accidents that previously could have been avoided.

Other conditions which reduce mobility in the elderly and are common enough when considering ageing in general terms are obesity, painful feet, poor sight, degenerative joint disease and respiratory disease. If health education and regular medical check-ups were more widely available they could alleviate many of these conditions.

3 *Internal organs*

The heart. In normal senescence the heart alters very little, although the muscles may weaken slightly and the beats show some irregularity. The heart muscle can enlarge (hypertrophy) to cope with the extra output needed to overcome oxygen deficiency in chronic respiratory disease or the reduced blood flow of arteriosclerosis.

The lungs. Lung capacity decreases with age due to a loss of elasticity in the lung tissue and the muscles used in respiration weaken. Chronic lung disease is so common, particularly in urban areas, that to a lay person it might be considered a normal result of ageing. The effect of diminished respiratory capacity, for whatever reason, may not be as debilitating in the elderly as in a younger person, for the slower movements of the older person need less oxygen. However, in times of stress the body requirements will be greater and there may be insufficient oxygen to supply the vital organs, particularly the brain.

The kidneys. The power of the kidneys to concentrate and excrete urine decreases with old age. The specific gravity of the urine of elderly people is rarely more than 1020, which is one reason why it is important for elderly people to drink plenty of fluids in order that there is sufficient solvent to encourage the excretion of waste products, especially protein (e g urea), to prevent their accumulation in the bloodstream. The renal threshold for sugar is frequently higher in older people than is normal (180 mg per 100 ml blood) for younger adults. Thus an elderly patient may be a diabetic without having glycosuria and so testing her urine for sugar is not sufficiently reliable. If diabetes is suspected, a glucose tolerance test will be performed (see Chapter 4).

Digestion and bowel function. The senses of taste and smell are often impaired in old age so that food is less appetising. Ill-fitting dentures or bad teeth make chewing difficult and eating loses much of its pleasure. The stomach lining atrophies and secretion of gastric juices and hydrochloric acid are diminished. This may cause indigestion or in more extreme cases may lead to pernicious anaemia (see Chapter 4). Weakened muscles in the alimentary canal may slow peristalsis but most of the complaints of indigestion and constipation in elderly people are likely to be due to an unsuitable diet and insufficient fluids.

Diet is discussed more fully in Chapter 7 and constipation in Chapter 4.

4 *The special senses*

Impairment of the senses of sight, hearing, taste, smell and touch are frequently found to some degree in old people and are important considerations when assessing the ability of the person to live independently.

Sight. Most people become long-sighted as they get older because the lens is less able to adjust to focus on near objects, a condition known as presbyopia. Unfortunately, many elderly people do not realise just how poor their sight is and have managed for years to 'get around' but at great risk to themselves, as for instance when crossing the road. Some may wear spectacles that were prescribed for them many years ago, which besides being scratched and dirty, are no longer suitable for their present eyesight. Others may wear spectacles not even prescribed for them but borrowed from a relative.

Ideally, all elderly people should attend an optician every two years. For those with a supplementary pension no charge is made for new glasses, and in many areas an optician will call at home. Refraction, however, requires the cooperation of the patient and it may be difficult to test the sight of a mildly confused person.

With ageing, the ability to distinguish colours and the speed with which the eye accommodates to light may be affected.

Large-print books are available from public libraries for those with poor sight and some people manage to read with the aid of a hand magnifying-glass. Elderly people who go blind late in life usually manage to remain reasonably independent in familiar surroundings and while they may not have the stamina to learn to read Braille or Moon they will enjoy the radio or the Talking Book service which is supplied by the Royal National Institute for the Blind. It has been noticed that many blind people accept their disability equably and do not show the frustrations of elderly deaf people.

Hearing. Most elderly people have some degree of hearing loss, especially of very high pitched sounds, which may be due to atrophy of the nervous tissue or disease of the bones in the middle ear (otosclerosis). The degree of hearing loss seems to depend on the volume and pitch of noise to which a person has been subjected during her working life, so that those who have spent their lives working in a noisy factory are frequently deaf to certain sounds from an early age. It is interesting to note that while some degree of deafness is accepted as a normal part of ageing in Western society, African tribesmen from a relatively noise-free environment have been found to have perfect hearing in old age.

Excessive wax in the external auditory meatus is a common cause of deafness in elderly people and the insertion of oily drops followed by syringing the ears may be ordered by the doctor to improve some long-standing deafness.

Talking to deaf people and hearing aids are discussed more fully in Chapter 6.

Young deaf people learn to lip read, and their other senses become more acute to compensate for their loss of hearing; elderly people on the other hand may withdraw from society as they become increasingly deaf and suspicious of what people are saying about them. Curiously, blindness arouses compassion and sympathy in most people but deaf people are often ridiculed or ignored.

Smell and taste. Sensory loss of smell and taste has already been mentioned under 'digestion'. Loss of smell is particularly dangerous for those elderly people who use gas and may fail to notice when it is leaking or has not ignited.

Touch, pain and the sensation of heat and cold. Loss of the sense of touch is usually minimal in old age. Awareness of pain varies very much with the pain threshold and mental state of the individual. The loss of sensation of heat and cold occurs in the extremities, particularly in the feet, due to their poor blood supply. This may lead to accidental burns from hot water bottles and fires. Equally, an elderly person may be unaware of the cold, which is usually gauged by the sensation felt in the fingers and toes.

Mental changes

Slowing of physical activity and impairment of the senses in elderly people does not imply a slowing and impairment of mental function. Many young people unfortunately seem to expect their elderly relatives to be of limited intelligence or 'senile', and this may account for the mishandling of elderly people by their children and other relatives. The word 'senile' has come to mean, in lay terms, a state of being old with implied mental confusion. Senile dementia as a medical term was a convenient label for an elderly person who showed signs of confusion, dementia or aggression, and once so labelled the patient and relatives could expect only custodial care in an institution.

Modern knowledge and understanding shows the causes of mental disorders in the elderly to be very varied. Elderly people are more likely to suffer from functional mental illness – depression and neurosis – than any other age group and many physical illnesses cause temporary mental impairment (see Chapter 4).

Intelligence. The peak of learning ability is considered to be reached in the early 20s. However, learning and memory are only two facets of intelligence; understanding and experience increase with age and are important intellectual resources in older people. To maintain a high level of mental ability the brain must be constantly stimulated and people who have been manual workers all their lives do not have the same resources to rely on in retirement as do professional people (see the following section on Retirement). Elderly people rarely find themselves over-taxing their intelligence but where there is a slowing of the mental processes those who live a physically active and pleasurable existence are more able to accept their mental limitations.

Memory. Long before old age memory, especially short-term memory for names and numbers, may begin to fail; short-term memory is important if a person is going to lead an independent life. The power to recall events long past is one of the characteristics of old age, as is repetitious, anecdotal conversation, but may be the effect of boredom, loneliness and lack of stimulation and should not be considered an inevitable part of growing old.

Intolerance. Elderly people often appear intolerant of new ideas or to changes in their way of life. They tend to adhere to a routine and may expect their relatives to conform to their habits. Such behaviour may be the only way elderly people can cope with the increased pace of life about them and their own failing mobility, impaired senses and slower reactions.

Character changes. Some elderly people seem to become more irritable, querulous and aggressive, and such behaviour may be thought of as characteristic of old age. While some people do behave in an anti-social way, it is likely that such behaviour has been with them throughout their life and that these traits become more noticeable in old age when they are dependent on others. It may happen that a daughter is oversolicitious in caring for her elderly mother who, becoming frustrated because she can no longer be independent, may respond by being awkward and demanding. When admitted to hospital she may be allowed more independence and sometimes her behaviour will improve, much to the distress of her caring daughter. Such a situation needs tactful handling, especially as the old lady will probably revert to her former ways when she returns home.

Extreme character changes are likely to be a sign of a pathological condition, such as cerebral ischaemia, and should not be accepted as part of growing old.

Social changes
Retirement from work at a fixed age with the right to a pension may at first sight be an ideal of any civilised society

but, in fact, it raises problems of adjustment which have only recently been recognised. Although people are retiring at an increasingly early age, retirement is still regarded as being the onset of old age, despite the fact that many retired people show none of the accepted signs of ageing.

Retirement brings about three major changes in a person's life:
1. reduced income (see Chapter 3);
2. increased leisure – with less money to spend;
3. loss of a job, which implies loss of status within the community, as well as loss of companionship and interests.

Men who have been in labouring or semi-skilled jobs are those who tend to find the effect of retirement the most devastating; unlike women, they do not usually have the running of the home to fill their time. While professional people may have developed other interests and hobbies with which to occupy themselves, the manual worker will more often resort to passive entertainments, such as watching television. Some reject their former workmates because they have not the money to join in communal entertainments. Few have prepared themselves to fill the extra hours and although some may be able to find part-time work, in times of high unemployment opportunities for the retired are few.

Awareness of the problems of adapting to retirement have led some firms, local authorities, and adult education centres to run pre-retirement courses. These usually consist of weekly talks and discussions on such topics as health, budgeting, welfare services available and ways of filling leisure time. The classes are not compulsory but inevitably the people most likely to attend are those least in need because they have recognised the problem. Nevertheless, these courses should be encouraged and extended as a preventive service.

Every old person needs a purpose in life, or a rôle to fulfil, whether it be caring for a spouse or as secretary of the local Darby and Joan Club. In the extended family of Victorian and Edwardian times, the grandparents, particularly the grandmother, were usually regarded as the centre of family activity and a source of advice and help with the younger children. While many grandparents still find great pleasure in their grandchildren, few actually live with them. With today's smaller families and many grandmothers still working, most grandchildren have grown up by the time the grandmother has the leisure to look after them. Labour saving devices mean that there is less work for them to do around the house and so the traditional rôle of the grandparent has diminished, leaving a gap not easily filled by clubs and community activities.

It can be strongly argued that education in the use of leisure time (which is increasing for the working adult, too) must start at school so that people regard leisure time and retirement as important a part of life as their time spent at work. However, until pensions bear more relation to wages, activity in retirement is likely to be curtailed by a lack of money.

Disengagement is a term which has been used to describe the very old person's process of detaching herself from involvement in active life. As a retired person grows older she can no longer keep pace, physically or mentally, with the changes about her; indeed, she has no need to. Withdrawing from everyday involvement leaves more time for reading and reflection on life and death. Such a state accounts for the serenity of some very elderly people who have come to terms with their age and limitations. In contrast there are those who fight to ward off the effects of old age, often with unhappy results, leaving them embittered and misunderstood by those about them.

Death. Few old people will talk about their own death. Some say they want to die but this may be a wish to escape from the unpleasantness of their present life. Those with strong religious convictions are probably able to face death more easily and will find comfort in talking to their priest or minister. Others, with the prospect of death close to them, may seek religious support in which previously they showed little interest.

Elderly people may be apprehensive, and many frightened, by the prospect of death and some may welcome the chance of talking, even in an oblique way, of their fears. It takes counselling skill to be able to listen sympathetically and without embarrassment to someone talking about death. A nurse who finds herself in this position must never dismiss the subject with some attempt at reassuring the patient she will not die (dying is discussed further in Chapter 6).

For Further Reading

Bromley, D. B. *The Psychology of Human Ageing*. Penguin Books, 1966
Ingleby, B. & Yorath, M. *Living With Old Age*. Hale, 1976

3. The Elderly Within the Community

It is easy for the nurse in a geriatric ward to think of her patients as existing only within the hospital walls, particularly if their stay has been long and there appears to be little chance of their returning home. However, it is important to remember that old people have a life and circle of friends and relatives outside the hospital and it is useful to know something of these to understand and to help each patient to the best advantage.

The social worker will have compiled a report on the patient's background: the sort of home she has, the facilities within the home, the extent of contact with neighbours and friends and what services are already provided (see Chapter 9). It is important, too, to know how the patient (and her relatives) feel about her returning home. As has already been stressed, geriatric medicine is both social as well as clinical and the physical condition of patients cannot be treated without due regard to the social situation to which they will return.

Unfortunately, it is all too easy to generalise when considering the elderly within the community. Statisticians and others accept the age of retirement – 65 for men and 60 for women – as being the onset of old age but an examination of people at this age will show that many have no signs of biological ageing other than some weakening of their physical powers. Despite this, society categorises people as old age pensioners, senior citizens, or simply the elderly and, although they are entitled to pensions and other benefits, such a label sets them apart from friends, neighbours and the people with whom they have been working.

Grouping people as an economic entity is a short step to treating them as a group in other respects. Some of the changes which occur as a result of ageing (outlined in the previous chapter) will appear in some people of retiring age to a greater or lesser degree, but it is a mistake to think of elderly people as being difficult, senile or forgetful. A nurse whose main experience of elderly people will be within an institution may readily endorse this attitude, yet a quick glance at some of the great statesmen, musicians and philosophers of history will show that man's mind can be as active and original in old age as at any other time. There is truth in the saying that a person is as old as he behaves and while some people are 'elderly' at 65, others are physically and mentally alert at 95. It is probable that people who show difficult character traits in old age may have had them all their lives, but it is only when they are dependent upon others that these traits become apparent.

What sort of a group are these 'Old Age Pensioners' within our society?

Population changes

Firstly, the elderly form an increasingly large proportion of the population. In 1870, in England and Wales, the proportion of the population over 65 was 5 per cent.; in 1974 it was 16·4 per cent. and this proportion is projected to rise to 17·4 per cent. in 1981 and then fall to 15·9 per cent. in 2001.* This means that at present about one in every six persons is over 65, although in some areas, such as the South Coast resorts, this ratio may rise to one in two or three persons, while conversely, in some of the new towns the proportion will be much lower. The increase in the actual numbers and in the proportion of elderly people to the total population is due to two main factors: (i) the increase in life expectancy, and (ii) the decrease in the size of families since the middle of the last century. In 1900 a one-year-old boy could expect to live to 52, while a one-year-old girl could expect to live to 54. In 1973, a year-old boy's life expectancy was 69 and a girl's was 75. This increase in life expectancy can be explained by the great improvements in public health and medical care during the last 70 years. The present generation of elderly people are the last of the large

---

* Social Trends: No 6. 1975 H M S O.

Victorian and Edwardian families and the significant decrease in the size of families since the beginning of this century is due mainly to economic reasons and to the greater acceptance of birth control.

Incomes and pensions

Secondly, of this large proportion of the population over 65, few will have a job and many will depend on the state contributory pension for an income. This age group will also make the greatest demands on the medical services as well as being the group most needing the social services, such as home helps. All these services are financed out of taxes and rates paid almost entirely by those who are working. Thus the elderly, like children, are dependent to a considerable degree upon those who are still working and of the two dependent groups, the children, upon whom the future of the country depends, are less likely to suffer if this support is curtailed. An attempt has been made through the Graduated Pension Scheme to fix the state pension on a scale appropriate to the wages earned but with inflation this is unlikely to provide an adequate income throughout the pensioner's life. Today, many retired people have to rely on a supplementary pension (formerly National Assistance) because the state contributory pension is insufficient to cope with high rents and heating costs. To many people the complexities of the forms required for the various supplementary benefits deter them from applying and others would rather struggle on with an inadequate income than accept what they regard as state 'charity'.

Those fortunate enough to have superannuation pensions are unlikely to get more than one half to two thirds of their final salary and although these schemes are becoming more widespread, a minority of people benefit in the present retired age group. In some cases the pension is so small that it does little to benefit the individual and yet prevents him from applying for social security supplementary pensions and associated benefits. Yet job pensions have a status and many elderly people are proud of the few pounds or pence a week they receive in recognition of their long service with a firm.

The over 65s include among them a significant group whose

income is barely adequate for their needs. The plight of these people is becoming better recognised and charities for housing and welfare not only help individuals but bring pressure for improvements to bear on local and central government. Even those who are not technically poor face a considerable drop in their income on retirement for which they have to make adjustments as well as come to terms with a pension continually decreasing in value as long as the cost of living rises ahead of, and disproportionate to, the rise in state pensions and wages.

Housing

Thirdly, for elderly people to remain in the community they not only need an adequate income but suitable housing. Many elderly people live in homes which are unsatisfactory for a variety of reasons. A few will live in the large family home which is now too big for their needs but where they must remain for lack of an acceptable alternative. Such houses are often old, in poor repair and expensive to heat and maintain. In some areas the local authority will buy such a house and offer to move the owner into somewhere more suitable. One of the problems of moving someone out of a family home is that modern dwellings are often too small for much of the large furniture old people have accumulated and, understandably, they are loath to part with it. The legal and financial complications of moving are often a deterrent to giving up an old house.

Other elderly people may be the long-term tenants of council or privately-rented property and this, too, may be unsuitably big or up several flights of stairs. While a council tenant may be able to transfer to other, more suitable accommodation so that the space may be used more economically, private tenants often have little choice of alternative accommodation. Many people will put up with the disadvantages of unsuitable accommodation rather than move away from the area they have known for a long time and from friends upon whom they rely. This is borne out in sociological studies of new towns. Some old people have even moved back to their old homes because they are unable to settle in the new, where facilities are more spread out and the close-knit circle of relatives and friends no longer exists.

In many urban areas there are still distressingly large numbers of elderly people living in very poor rented accommodation, where they may have lived for many years paying a low (controlled) rent. Such places are usually multi-occupied, with an outside lavatory or one shared by several tenants, and there is rarely a bathroom. Despite the fact that some controlled rents have been phased out by recent legislation, the low income from places like these plus the uncertainty of the future of the area may mean that the landlord is disinclined to improve or even maintain his property. The elderly person 'puts up with it' because there is no alternative and council waiting lists are long, with insufficient accommodation suitable for elderly people.

Some people, about the time of their retirement, choose to move away from the area where they have lived and worked for much of their lives to the seaside or country. Towns on the East and South Coasts and in North Wales and on the Lancashire coast have a very high proportion of retired people living in communities of bungalows on the outskirts of the towns. While such a move may have many advantages for the newly retired, if circumstances change for the worse elderly neighbours can offer little support and great demands are made on the local authority services. These relative newcomers are difficult for the local authority to re-house and while some, on the death of a partner, may return to their original area where they still have friends, others continue to live on in a state of great isolation and poverty. People moving out of large urban areas often idealise their new surroundings and fail to realise that such essentials as shops and hospitals are often far away and that public transport is poor.

In the past one of the children – usually a daughter – would forgo marriage in order to stay at home to look after the elderly parents. Although this does still happen, living patterns have changed in recent years and society has become more mobile. Fifty years ago children would probably settle near their parents' home and marry someone met locally, whereas today young people are likely to move all over the country in search of jobs. Within large, nationwide and international companies promotion may even depend upon moving to another part of the country and the elderly parent is unlikely to be willing to move, too, even if accommodation is available.

At one time the old people's home, either managed by the local authority or by a private organisation, was thought to be the best solution for those elderly people who, for one reason or another, could no longer live independently. Yet to many old people the idea of such a home is reminiscent of the old workhouses, which were still in use as late as the 1920's and, indeed, many of the first local authority homes provided under Part III of the National Assistance Act (1948) necessarily used the original workhouse buildings. Even the newer, smaller purpose-built homes have tended to become a refuge for extremely infirm elderly people who need a great deal of supervision, and this is not the ideal alternative accommodation sought by people, mentally and physically able, who find their house too large, or their flat just too high. Many elderly people would rather struggle on in their own homes than risk losing their independence and privacy in an institution.

The present trend represents a reversion to a time before the workhouse became the last resort for the elderly poor. The idea of sheltered accommodation in warden-supervised flatlets or bungalows is a development of the almshouses still in use in some villages and older towns. These units, which should be built at the centre of the village or housing estate and close to shops and buses, allow the elderly person to remain independent and to keep some of her personal possessions while living in a home which she can manage within her income and with the knowledge that help is readily available. Sadly, the need for such accommodation at present far outnumbers the places actually available.

Loneliness

Fourthly, in this age group there will be many people living alone. A minority of these will be well adjusted to their situation and have a wide circle of friends and a variety of interests. Others, particularly the recently bereaved, find living alone difficult to accept and complain of loneliness and a fear of being by themselves. Few people are prepared for the time when they are suddenly left alone and there is a high incidence of illness and falls among those who have had a recent bereavement. Apart from actually being alone, women often have to contend with new and confusing financial responsibilities and a reduced income.

Many widows and widowers will refuse offers to live with their children for fear of being a burden, a fact that is often forgotten by those who criticise the children for neglecting their parents. Even some elderly people living with their families complain of loneliness because they have moved away from the area and the friends they have known.

While old people's clubs, adult education classes and other social groups may provide a new interest for some lonely people, for others, group socialising is abhorrent and it would be a grave mistake to force someone into group activities. Aids to combat loneliness include a radio or television, a library service and voluntary agencies who provide a regular visitor prepared to build up an effective relationship with the lonely person. Occasionally an elderly person will withdraw completely from society and become a recluse, refusing help and neglecting herself. On very rare occasions a person may be admitted to a mental hospital, either voluntarily or under Section 25 of the Mental Health Act, 1959 (Compulsory Admission). Others will continue to exist almost unknown to their neighbours until they succumb to an illness and are found dead in their homes days or weeks later. While it is easy to criticise relatives, neighbours and the statutory services for allowing such a situation to arise, it is the right of everyone to live, within reason, as they choose and this right must be respected.

Vulnerability within the community

Finally, the elderly as a group are particularly vulnerable in a society which in some respects they have 'outgrown'. In the last 50 years the pace of life has increased as never before and for people whose mental and physical speed is slowing as part of a natural process, the strain of keeping abreast of present day changes can be overwhelming. For instance, the speed and volume of traffic today can terrify elderly people whose vision and hearing may be impaired and evidence of their vulnerability is shown in the figures of accidents involving pedestrians where the elderly and children are by far the largest number of people involved. Ironically, the increase in the number of private cars has meant a decrease in local bus and train services and the first to suffer are the elderly people, of a generation that may never have needed to drive a car. Such people lose their highly-valued independence and become reliant upon neighbours and relatives to ferry them about or do their shopping.

Money is another aspect of modern life which elderly people frequently find difficult to manage. They do not understand inflation and when they find prices higher than they remember they feel they are being cheated – and it may be that some unscrupulous people do exploit their vulnerability. Decimalisation still confuses some elderly people who are slow to work out change and the relative cost of items. Many, too, find the large impersonal supermarkets physically and mentally exhausting and will do their shopping in smaller local shops where goods are likely to be more expensive. Heating and lighting are essential for elderly people, but with a barely adequate income these are the items that may be curtailed. This inevitable economy can lead to accidental hypothermia, or falls as a result of poor lighting.

The television, which today is taken so much for granted, can be of great benefit to an elderly person but its portrayal of violence and of sexual scenes unmentionable in former times can cause an elderly person distress and insecurity, especially if they have led a sheltered life. It is extremely important to understand the anxieties of elderly people living in the modern world and to realise that, trivial as they may seem, no amount of reassurance is going to change long-held beliefs and a need to cling to the past.

All is not as gloomy as this chapter may imply. The vast majority (94 per cent.) of elderly people live in the community outside any institution, and most live independently and cope adequately. Those who are admitted to hospital are among the minority who can no longer cope, whether temporarily or permanently, because of illness. Understanding the background to this breakdown will go a long way to understanding the patient herself. Today the community can offer more and more support for the elderly and the services available are discussed in Chapter 9; there is a growing awareness of the problems and needs of elderly people and over recent years a number of pressure groups, such as Age Concern and Help the Aged, have concerned themselves with improving the quality of life of the elderly within the community. These charities will often call upon local resources through old people's welfare committees and it is at this level that Good Neighbour schemes and voluntary helpers reach the individual. Young people, particularly, are often involved in local Task Forces and similar voluntary agencies to help the elderly and often there is a feeling of greater accord between these age groups than between adjacent generations. These services are not only invaluable for maintaining elderly people within the community but are essential for supporting people newly discharged from hospital.

For Further Reading

Pilch, M.(Ed). *The Retirement Book*. Hamish Hamilton, 1974
Townsend, P. *The Family Life of Old People*. Penguin Books, 1963
Townsend, P. & Wedderburn, D. *The Aged in the Welfare State*. G. Bell & Sons, 1966
Tunstall, J. *Old and Alone*. Routledge & Kegan Paul, 1966

4. The Diseases and Hazards of Old Age

Introduction
The predominating causes of ill-health in old age are the degenerative conditions, mental disorders and inadequate social support. It is the treatment of these conditions, and the preventive aspects of specific hazards, which distinguishes geriatric medicine from the medical care of adults of middle-age in whom the diseases of stress – myocardial infarction, hypertension and so on – and the malignant diseases are more common. The scope of this book is limited and only the conditions most frequently encountered in the geriatric department are discussed here. Treatment of the disorders has intentionally been kept very general and specific drugs and their dosages have not usually been included as these will vary with individual patients and with the doctor prescribing them. A list of books for further reading about specific conditions and drugs is included at the end of this chapter.

Characteristics of disease in the elderly
1. **Multiple pathology.** Elderly people commonly suffer from more than one condition at a time because degeneration, failure or infection involving one or more of the body's systems has a widespread effect throughout the other systems. For example:

'Mrs H., aged 78 years, was admitted with an acute exacerbation of her long-standing chronic bronchitis. Upon examination she was found to be in cardiac failure because her respiratory infection is making excessive demands upon her heart. She is also anaemic and has varicose ulcers; the anaemia is a contributory cause of her cardiac failure. Treatment of her bronchitis and anaemia will improve the cardiac output and the improved circulation will hasten the healing of the varicose ulcers.'

It is important to understand the relationship between the systems of the body and how, in old age, the balance between them can become very precarious.

2. Degenerative conditions. Degenerative conditions are by definition found more commonly in the elderly and they occur as the result of stress over many years which alters the structure of the organs involved. Degeneration is a pathological rather than a physiological ageing (see Chapter 2), although it may be difficult to decide which process is involved in some conditions very common in the aged, such as increasing deafness. Degenerative conditions, such as atherosclerosis, osteoarthritis and chronic bronchitis, play a major part in the disease pattern of the elderly, and while not usually the immediate cause of admission to hospital, the presence of one or more of these conditions may greatly influence the patient's prognosis.

3. Malignant disease. Elderly patients do suffer from neoplastic diseases but a slowing down of cell growth means that malignant growths develop less rapidly and many can be treated successfully with radiotherapy or surgery. Secondary growths can occur many years after a primary growth has apparently been successfully treated and this may cause difficulty in diagnosis.

4. Confusional states. One of the first signs of physical illness in the elderly can be a change in their mental alertness. It should not be assumed that signs of confused behaviour, forgetfulness or increased aggressiveness are due to senility and an underlying cause must always be sought.(see page 53). Elderly people suffer from affective disorders, such as depression and anxiety, and behavioural changes will occur as in other age groups (see page 55).

5. Iatrogenic disorders. A condition that occurs as the result of the treatment the patient has been prescribed is called an iatrogenic disorder. Elderly people particularly are susceptible to the side effects of certain drugs and with an ever increasing number of drugs being prescribed there is a real danger of their taking the wrong medicine or dosage. The barbiturates, notably, cause confusion in this age group and are rarely prescribed now, but drugs for Parkinsonism (such as orphenadrine) can also cause confusional states. Hypotensive drugs may cause a sudden and dangerous fall in the blood pressure and even a mild sedative drug may induce a deep sleep that causes an old person to be incontinent or confused.

The onset of confusion in a previously alert patient may be the first sign of the adverse effect of a drug and the nurse's careful observation of any change in the patient's behaviour and its time of onset can help the doctor in his diagnosis and treatment.

6. Signs and symptoms. Elderly people have difficulty in describing their symptoms and they may have such a multiplicity of complaints that the most predominant condition at the time may become all important. Deafness or confusion will make history-taking more difficult and the doctor must rely extensively for his diagnosis on his clinical examination and tests, on the observations of the nursing staff and on any help he may obtain from relatives.

The normal body temperature of an elderly person is usually lower than that of a younger adult and does not always rise in response to infection. A rise in the pulse and respiratory rates are more reliable guides to the presence of an acute infection.

Hypothermia, a fall in the body temperature, is a dangerous condition in elderly people (see page 60). Ideally all geriatric patients should have their temperature taken rectally with a low-reading thermometer ($22 \cdot 8°C$ ($75°F$)) on admission to hospital. Every nurse must be aware of the dangers of a patient becoming hypothermic, even in a well heated hospital ward.

Pain is a complex symptom to assess in the elderly as many have learnt to live with the chronic pain of, for instance, arthritis and appear to tolerate pain which would be unacceptable to a younger person. Typically, a myocardial infarction, which in a younger adult causes an acute, severe pain, may be passed off as an attack of indigestion in the older patient. Patients often do not feel pain where the blood supply is poor, as for example around pressure sores and ulcers. In contrast, an elderly person may react to pain in a manner which is out of all proportion to the severity of the condition, because she is confused, emotionally labile or wanting to draw attention to herself, reactions which themselves give some indication of the patient's mental state.

SECTION 1. PHYSICAL DISEASES OF THE ELDERLY

1. Diseases of the nervous system

Cerebro-vascular disease

A cerebro-vascular accident occurs when the blood supply to part of the brain is cut off, causing a temporary or permanent ischaemia. Patients suffering from cerebro-vascular disorders are commonly seen in geriatric wards and strokes are responsible for many of the handicaps suffered by elderly people.

Atherosclerosis. The arteries of the brain are particularly susceptible to a degenerative process known as atherosclerosis where there is a loss of elasticity in the walls of the arteries, and plaques of fatty tissue (atheroma) are deposited on the walls within the lumen of the vessels. The blood supply to the brain would be more affected by atherosclerosis but for the system of interconnecting arteries, principally at the Circle of Willis, which allows a colateral circulation to take over if one artery is blocked.

Transient ischaemic attacks. Transient ischaemic attacks will sometimes herald a complete stroke and are called a 'stroke in evolution'. They occur over a period and are caused by a temporary reduction in the blood supply to part of the brain due to illness or to a fall in blood pressure from shock or from the effect of certain drugs. The patient may complain of temporary weakness or blurred vision and may become mildly confused, occasionally being left with a slight residual weakness which can become more disabling with each attack.

Strokes. Strokes are defined as cerebral damage which manifests itself for more than 24 hours. The causes of strokes are:

Cerebral thrombosis. A stroke caused by one of the cerebral arteries becoming blocked by a thrombus (blood clot) may be preceded by transient ischaemic attacks. The onset of a stroke caused by a cerebral thrombus is less dramatic than one caused by an embolism or haemorrhage (see below). The patient may find that one side of the body is weak or paralysed on attempting to get up in the morning or, on rising from sitting down, may collapse as a leg gives way.

The prognosis of a stroke caused by a cerebral thrombosis is usually quite good. After a time, the blood establishes a colateral circulation and the function of the affected limbs, particularly the lower limb, will improve with physiotherapy. There is always the risk of another thrombus forming.

Cerebral embolism. An embolism consists of a portion of blood clot, atheroma or vegetation which becomes detached from the site of origin and travels in the bloodstream until it blocks an arterial vessel. A cerebral embolism causing a stroke by occluding one of the cerebral arteries is likely to arise from the thrombosed area of the wall of the left ventricle following an old cardiac infarction. The patient will suddenly lose consciousness. The size of the embolism and the affected area of the brain will decide the extent of the paralysis and the prognosis. There is always the risk of further emboli occurring.

Cerebral haemorrhage. Haemorrhage into the brain from a burst artery is the most serious form of stroke and the mortality is high. It is more likely to occur in patients with hypertension. The onset is sudden and dramatic and, depending on the severity and the site of the haemorrhage, the patient can be comatosed for several days; damage to the brain tissue may be so severe that death is inevitable. The physical effects of the stroke will lessen if pressure from the cerebral oedema subsides as blood is re-absorbed, but the residual damage depends on the site of the lesion and is often very severe.

Pseudobulbar palsy. Cerebrovascular accidents which affect both sides of the brain, or localised atherosclerosis near the brain stem and basal ganglia, can cause this condition. Apart from paralysis or paresis (weakness) of the skeletal muscles on both sides of the body, paralysis of the pharyngeal muscles will cause difficulty in swallowing and there is a serious risk that the patient will inhale food or fluid. Speech will be slurred and the patient may become very emotional, crying and laughing without cause.

The effects of a cerebro-vascular accident

The effects of a stroke can be very varied, from mild to very severe. There is often a mixture of muscle weakness, sensory loss and intellectual damage.

Hemiplegia is the complete paralysis of the skeletal muscles on one side of the body due to damage to the motor nerve fibres in the brain which control their movement. The affected side will be opposite to that of the damaged cerebral hemisphere as the motor nerve pathways cross in the medulla. Depending on the site of the lesion, only a partial hemiplegia may be present, e g paralysis of one arm. **Hemiparesis** is a weakness rather than a paralysis of one side.

Speech disorders. Dysphasia is the term used to describe the distressing effects of a stroke if the speech centre is affected, the patient being unable to understand or use language. Sensory dysphasia is the inability to understand what is said or written and motor dysphasia is the inability to express in words what is understood. Both forms of dysphasia may occur together. Thus a patient may find the simplest command incomprehensible and her replies to questions, even if she does understand, may be bizarre or the complete opposite to what is intended. **Aphasia** is a total loss of speech.

A patient whose ability to communicate is affected should be treated with great understanding and patience. A patient with motor dysphasia may be able to understand quite well what is being said but as her replies are incoherent she may be thought to be confused, which can only add to her frustration. The degree of a patient's understanding may be gauged by her response to simple commands, a look of understanding in her eyes and facial expression as well as obvious gestures such as a nod or a shake of the head. Treatment is discussed under Speech Therapy (Chapter 8).

Dysarthria is a mechanical disorder of speech which may follow a stroke or occur in Parkinson's disease or in pseudobulbar palsy. If the muscles used in the production of speech – those of the larynx, pharynx and the facial muscles – are affected the patient will have difficulty in articulating words although she will be able to understand what is said. Speech therapy can help this condition.

Mental disturbances. Apart from the physical effects and impaired comprehension following a stroke, a patient's recovery may be delayed by a poor short-term memory or difficulty in concentration for any length of time. She may deny that she is paralysed or neglect the affected side as though it were no part of her – a condition known as **anosognosia.**

A patient may become **emotionally labile** following a stroke, crying at the slightest cross word or past memory, laughing incongruously in conversation. It can be very disturbing for the relatives who need to be told that it is a consequence of the stroke and is best quietly accepted without comment until the moment of tears or laughter is passed. True depression, which can hinder rehabilitation unless it is recognised and treated, may also follow a stroke. Anxiety may also develop, the patient losing all confidence and literally trembling with fear when any attempt is made to encourage self help and increase mobility.

Visual defects. Homonymous hemianopia, the loss of the visual field on one side only in both eyes, may occur. This may not be apparent to the patient who can see directly ahead, but a nurse or relative standing to one side may realise that the patient is unaware of her presence. It is important that a patient with hemianopia should always be approached from her 'good' side and that lockers and chairs for visitors are also placed on that side.

The nursing care of a patient with a stroke

A patient may be unconscious for two or three days following a stroke and the length of the unconscious period is an indication of the severity of the stroke. During this time the nursing care is all important. The patient should be maintained and nursed in a semi-prone position in order to keep the air passages clear and allow secretions to drain from the mouth. The patient should be turned regularly at two-hourly intervals, great care being taken to position the limbs suitably to prevent deformities. Contractures occur as the result of muscular spasm holding a joint in flexion; eventually it will become fixed unless the joint is put through its full range of movements two or three times a day. The affected arm should be supported on a pillow with the shoulder abducted and the elbow slightly flexed in a position which will be of the greatest use to the patient should there be some residual paralysis. A splint under the wrist and forearm will prevent wrist drop and a rolled bandage or a soft ball in the palm of the hand will help to prevent the fingers from becoming clawed.

To prevent permanent contractures of the knee joint, it may be necessary for the patient to wear a splint behind the knee for short periods. Foot drop must be prevented by placing the feet against a firm pillow or foam pad, supported by a foot board so that the feet are at right angles to the legs (dorsiflexed) and not extended (plantarflexed). Great care must be taken to ensure that pressure sores do not develop under the splints and in the particularly vulnerable areas – the heels, elbows, sacrum and hips.

If the patient remains unconscious for more than 24 hours, some form of artificial feeding will be necessary; if a nasogastric tube is passed, it is *vital* to ensure that it is in the stomach (see p. 121). Alternatively, intravenous fluids may be given which must be calculated very accurately as too great a fluid intake can overload the circulation and precipitate cardiac failure.

Once conscious and able to sit up, the patient should be encouraged to do as much as possible for herself (which may be particularly difficult if the dominant side has been affected) by being shown how to lift and move any paralysed limbs, and to exercise fingers and wrist with the good hand. Inability to comprehend and communicate may make it very difficult for the patient to co-operate and the nursing staff must show great patience.

The physiotherapist will initiate a long-term programme of treatment (see Chapter 8) that patients and relatives will be able to continue at home. The type of exercise that patients can carry out will depend on the degree of recovery of movement, their mental state and any other disabling condition they may have, such as arthritis. Re-training patients whose comprehension and speech is impaired is a long task and may take several years. In some cases the patients are so disabled that they may have to spend the rest of their life in long-stay care (see Chapter 5).

Degenerative diseases
Parkinson's disease. Parkinson's disease is a degenerative condition of the brain which affects the basal ganglia; it is probably not one but several diseases which make up the typical picture of Parkinsonism. Whatever the cause in young adults, in old age Parkinsonism usually results from atherosclerosis.

The three features of Parkinsonism are rigidity, tremor and postural disturbances. The rigid muscles of the face form a blank, mask-like expression and the vocal cords are affected so that the voice lacks modulation and is similarly expressionless. The tremor is regular and can affect one or more limbs and the face. It is seen especially in the hands and can be controlled for short periods by voluntary effort; it will stop altogether when the patient is asleep but it will get worse if the old person is agitated. The gait is typical in that the patient may have difficulty initiating walking but once moving takes hurried, tiny steps without swinging the arms and appears to walk quickly to prevent toppling forwards. The rigidity and the fatiguability of the muscles may become so severe that old people suffering from this condition are unable to move their limbs without great effort and there is a danger that the joints will become permanently contracted.

The intellect of such patients is not usually affected but when they can no longer do much physically they may become withdrawn and passive. The blank, expressionless face and voice may give the impression of deeper withdrawal than is actually present and the nurse must try to assess the patient's true feelings.

The treatment of a patient with Parkinson's disease. Drug treatment will relieve some of the rigidity and tremor but there is no real cure for this degenerative condition. The drugs used to reduce the rigidity are benzhexol hydrochloride and orphenadrine, and anti-histamine drugs such as diphenhydramine may be used to reduce the tremor. L-Dopa is a newer drug which acts upon the signals that control muscular movement and may help to reduce the rigidity and fatiguability of the muscles, improve the tremor and generally increase mobility. Some of the drugs can cause temporary confusional states and have other serious side effects such as vomiting, depression or anxiety; the nurse must therefore be alert to any changes in the patient's behaviour after treatment with one of these drugs has been started.

Physiotherapy will be required to help patients to exercise their rigid limbs and to give them confidence in walking, perhaps with the help of a suitable walking frame. Old people who enjoy reading, television and radio will find it easier to accept their immobility than those who have led a more active life.

Dementia. Degeneration of nervous tissue in the brain gives rise to two distinctive types of dementia found in elderly people. These are discussed in the section, 'Mental Disorders', page 54.

2. Cardio-vascular disease

Many elderly people fear that they are suffering from 'heart trouble' or 'blood pressure', yet these conditions are not necessarily the direct cause of serious illness in old age. When caring for old people, this anxiety should not be aggravated by talk of 'cardiac disease' or 'high blood pressure' in a way that may be misinterpreted. To some people the word 'cardiac' alone signifies a 'bad heart' and misunderstandings can lead to an unnecessarily inactive life which in itself may worsen the situation by increasing the risk of obesity, thrombosis and pneumonia.

Pulse dysrythmias are common in old age and may cause needless anxiety. (*a*) *Palpitations* are usually caused by an extrasystole (premature beat) and have little significance. (*b*) *Paroxysmal tachycardia* (short periods of a rapid pulse rate) is also not usually indicative of serious heart disease but both these conditions are distressing and alarming for elderly patients. (*c*) *Atrial fibrillation* is more serious and is usually associated with ischaemic heart disease. The radial pulse is irregular as the ineffective contractions of the ventricles are not felt at the extremities and the apex beat is a better guide to the heart's regularity and strength. Atrial fibrillation is controlled by digitalis and counting of the apex and radial pulse rate simultaneously by two nurses at prescribed intervals is necessary to show a reduction in the pulse deficit and so indicate the effectiveness of the treatment. (*d*) *Coupling* or a pulse of two beats in rapid succession followed by a slight pause is a sign of digitalis poisoning (see page 35). (*e*) *Heart block* is also associated with ischaemic heart disease. Impulses from the atria fail to reach the ventricles which beat independently at a much slower rate. At times in unstable heart block insufficient blood is pumped to the brain and the patient becomes temporarily unconscious – an episode called a Stokes Adams attack. These attacks can occur so frequently that the patient may be confined to a chair, for fear of falling. A battery operated pacemaker can be inserted to stimulate the rate and rhythm of ventricular contractions.

Angina pectoris is associated with intermittent ischaemia of the heart muscle and, typically, is a severe pain in the centre of the chest radiating down the left arm and up into the throat and jaw. The onset usually occurs in middle age in people with a history of heart disease and hypertension. Such patients will learn to live with their angina and to know how active they can be without provoking an attack. The pain is controlled with glyceryl trinitrate tablets which are absorbed sublinguinally and are rapidly effective as they dilate the coronary arteries and so increase the blood supply to the myocardium. The severity of the attacks will normally lessen with old age as activity is reduced. Older people may think they have angina when all they are suffering from is indigestion or even a chest infection; again this may cause unnecessary anxiety.

Heart failure. The heart is said to be in failure when the blood pumped from ventricle either/or both is of insufficient volume to meet the body's requirements. As elderly people tend to lead a relatively restricted life they will make fewer demands upon their heart than would younger people. However, their cardiac reserve – that is, the ability of the heart to cope with any extra strain – is slight, so that they may fluctuate between having an adequate cardiac output and being in cardiac failure when extra demands are made upon the heart. Heart failure in the elderly is rarely due to a single cause but occurs when the heart, already damaged by ischaemia or valvular disease, has to cope with an added strain, such as anaemia, obesity, chest disease, hypertension or even unsuitable housing. Many elderly people live comfortably at home with incipient heart failure controlled by digoxin and a mild diuretic such as hydrochlorothiazide.

An early sign of heart failure in an elderly person may be

mild confusion or agitation due to cerebral hypoxia which will improve as the cardiac output increases and sufficient oxygen reaches the brain.

Ischaemic heart disease is the most common major cause of cardiac failure in the elderly. The coronary arteries that supply the muscles of the heart are particularly susceptible to atherosclerotic changes (see page 26) and while a younger person may suffer from a typical attack of myocardial infarction, the first signs of ischaemia of the heart muscle in an older person may be increasing evidence of heart failure, with dyspnoea, oedema and confusion. Atrial fibrillation is often present in ischaemic heart disease.

Pulmonary heart disease (Cor pulmonale) is the name given to failure of the right side of the heart which is the end of a sequence of events found in patients with chronic bronchitis. As the bronchioles become more blocked with mucus and scarred, the alveoli beyond become distended and filled with static gases. Damage to the capillaries surrounding the alveoli causes congestion in the pulmonary vessels which increase the pressure in the right ventricle. A patient with right ventricular failure due to pulmonary congestion will have central cyanosis, severe dyspnoea and a full, bounding pulse. Cerebral hypoxia may cause her to be confused and agitated.

Valvular heart disease. Damage to the mitral or aortic valve resulting from rheumatic fever in early life may have its effect in old age as an incompetent valve can be a contributory cause of left ventricular failure. Extra effort is needed by the myocardium to overcome the resistance of the damaged valve and eventually the increased back pressure of blood in the pulmonary veins causes congestion of the lungs. The patient will suffer from sudden attacks of severe dyspnoea and will cough up much watery sputum. People with severely damaged valves are unlikely to survive to old age, but many elderly people are found on admission to hospital to have some valvular damage, which in conjunction with another condition, such as anaemia, can precipitate cardiac failure.

Other causes of heart failure. Several other conditions such as anaemia (see page 45), hypertension (page 36) and thyrotoxicosis (page 51) predispose to heart failure; poor social conditions are another contributory factor.

The treatment of the patient with heart failure
Elderly people with heart failure will need rest but should not be totally confined to bed unless their condition has reached a terminal stage. They may feel more comfortable sitting in a high-backed arm chair with their legs supported on a footstool but they should be encouraged to stand and walk short distances each day.

Oxygen may be helpful if the patient is cyanosed and restless. It must be prescribed by the doctor and should be given in a low concentration (2–3 litres per minute) to prevent too much oxygen from entering the bloodstream and lowering the carbon dioxide level, so reducing the stimulus to respiration. Elderly patients do not easily tolerate the apparatus used for administering oxygen and a variety of methods may be tried, a nasal catheter or a ventimask usually being the most acceptable.

Drugs used in heart failure. *Digoxin* or other preparations of digitalis are usually prescribed for patients in heart failure and many elderly people have taken digoxin for years to control incipient heart failure. Digoxin acts upon the myocardium by strengthening it and by slowing the rate of ventricular contractions, thus improving the cardiac output. If atrial fibrillation is present the digoxin also acts on the bundle of His and between the sino-atrial node and atrio-ventricular node by slowing the rate of conduction of impulses, so improving the cardiac output by allowing the ventricles to fill before contracting.

The toxic effects of digitalis can be very serious particularly because the drug is accumulative and for this reason it may be prescribed for six days only each week. As each patient's sensitivity to digitalis is different, anyone newly given the drug must be closely observed. The patient's pulse must be taken before each dose to detect the presence of bradycardia (usually considered to be a pulse rate below 60 beats a minute) or of coupling of the beats, both of which are signs of digoxin poisoning. If either are present, the dose should be withheld and the doctor informed. Nausea, vomiting, dizziness, confusion and yellow vision can also occur in digoxin poisoning. It may be possible for the doctor to eliminate these effects by prescribing a different preparation of digitalis. The effectiveness of digoxin is increased when the level of potassium in the blood is low and potassium supplements are therefore necessary to prevent the heart becoming hypersensitive to digoxin, when it is given with diuretics, which deplete the body of potassium.

Diuretics are prescribed to increase the urinary output and reduce oedema. They are best given early in the morning so that the diuresis occurs during the daytime and the patient does not have a disturbed night. Diuretics can be given orally or by intramuscular injection. They may be given on alternate days or twice a week and it is important that they are given correctly as too frequent doses could cause the patient to become dehydrated, incontinent, or hypokalaemic.

Salt must be restricted in the diet as it increases fluid retention.

Hypertension. Many elderly people have a form of essential hypertension which, with a systolic pressure above 200 mg Hg and a raised diastolic pressure but no other symptoms, may only be discovered during an examination for an unrelated condition. Those particularly at risk are the obese, especially women, and those living under stress, which will include many elderly people. Prolonged hypertension speeds up the process of atherosclerosis, which in turn will contribute to a raised blood pressure. It will also cause hypertrophy and subsequent failure of the left ventricle, especially where there is ischaemia of the myocardium. If atherosclerosis is present there is also a greater risk of cardiac infarction and cerebral thrombosis, and hypertension is a precursor of renal failure.

Hypertension in elderly patients is seldom treated with hypotensive drugs as a sudden fall in blood pressure may precipitate a cerebro-vascular accident or other side-effects. Treatment may, however, be indicated when complications, such as retinopathy, renal failure, or cardiac failure are present, or when the diastolic pressure is persistently above 120 mg Hg. In most cases it is far better to encourage the patient to diet and as far as possible to relieve her stress. Cardiac failure occurring as the result of prolonged hypertension is treated like any other form of cardiac failure.

Peripheral vascular disease. Atherosclerosis affecting the arteries which supply the legs will mean that insufficient blood reaches the feet. The patient may first complain of numbness, 'pins and needles' or a cramp-like pain in the calf muscles known as intermittent claudication. The serious complication of arterial occlusion affecting the legs is gangrene.

Gangrene may first start as a small cut or sore on the foot – perhaps the result of inexpert treatment of a corn or a nick with the nail scissors. The area becomes a reddish, dusky colour, then black and necrotic. If a toe is affected it may separate from the foot. If the affected area becomes infected the gangrene will spread more quickly and the infection can become so severe that the patient dies of a generalised toxaemia. The pain associated with peripheral vascular disease can be severe, particularly at night. If gangrene has developed the actual lesion may not be painful, but the patient can suffer mental anguish both from the knowledge of existing gangrene and from the threat of amputation.

Treatment of the patient with peripheral vascular disease and gangrene. The patient who is known to suffer from peripheral vascular disease should be taught to take great care of her feet by wearing well fitting shoes and by always attending a chiropodist for foot care. Any small cut or sore on her feet should be treated by her doctor who may recommend daily dressing by the home nurse. The blood supply to the area must be maintained as far as possible by treating cardiac failure and anaemia if they arise. Bed rest is not indicated as it carries a risk of the patient developing pressure sores.

The circulation may be improved in younger, fitter patients with arterial surgery, involving either a by-pass graft or endarterectomy but where gangrene has developed amputation will usually be necessary, before the patient becomes seriously ill. Elderly people can be fitted with artificial limbs and acquire a reasonable mobility, or they may be able to retain their independence in a wheelchair. The success of rehabilitation after an amputation will depend largely upon the patient's ability to cope with psychological effects of losing a limb and the nursing staff can give a great deal of support to the patient both before and after the operation.

3. Chest diseases

Chest disease is so common in old age that some lay people accept it as a normal process of ageing. Age reduces the elasticity of the lungs and weakens the muscles of respiration so that the air intake is reduced and less oxygen reaches the blood. In normal circumstances this will be of little significance, the old people having a reduced need for oxygen because they are less active, but if chronic chest disease further reduces the amount of oxygen reaching the blood the balance between sufficiency and insufficiency becomes precarious.

Chronic bronchitis. Chronic bronchitis, colloquially known as the English Disease, is four times more common in men than in women. It occurs particularly in areas with a damp and polluted atmosphere and in people who smoke heavily and who are obese. Its onset is gradual, with repeated chesty colds or attacks of acute bronchitis, over several winters. The lining of the bronchioles becomes chronically inflamed (hypertrophied) and produces excessive quantities of frothy sputum which will reduce the respiratory process. For most of the year, the patient will be mildly dyspnoeic and will cough up watery sputum each morning, but any infection of the respiratory tract, such as a common cold or influenza, will exacerbate the condition into a state of acute bronchitis.

Acute bronchitis. Although acute bronchitis in elderly people usually occurs as an exacerbation of chronic bronchitis it may follow an attack of influenza or a cold in someone without a history of chronic chest disease. Because the elderly respond to an acute infection less dramatically than the young, without a rise in temperature, the first sign of acute bronchitis may be confused behaviour, which indicates a degree of cerebral hypoxia. The patient will become cyanosed, with a rapid respiration rate, will cough up thick, purulent sputum and may show signs of early cardiac failure.

Treatment of the patient with bronchitis. Acute bronchitis is treated with antibiotics and drugs to improve the cardiac output if heart failure is present (see page 33). Expectorants will help the patient to cough up the thick sputum, and a broncho-dilator, such as choline theophylinate, will relieve the spasm. After an acute attack the physiotherapist may help such patients to clear their lungs by means of postural drainage and breathing exercises.

Patients with chronic bronchitis may have an antibiotic prescribed for any cold or mild, upper respiratory tract infection to prevent acute bronchitis developing.

Emphysema. Emphysema is an advanced stage of chronic bronchitis when the bronchioles becomes so blocked that air can no longer freely enter the terminal bronchioles beyond. The alveoli lose their convoluted shape and become distended, fibrosed and filled with air, which also has difficulty in being expelled, therefore increasing the amount of dead air space in the lungs where no exchange of gases can take place. The distended alveoli cause the pressure in the pulmonary vessels surrounding them to rise which will cause extra strain on the right ventricle of the heart and eventually lead to right-sided heart failure (see pulmonary heart disease, page 34).

A patient with advanced emphysema will be very dyspnoeic and will only be able to live a restricted life. As the lungs are permanently damaged her condition will not improve but prophylactic antibiotics may be given to prevent further infection and damage.

Pneumonia. Pneumonia has been described as the 'old man's friend' because it is so often the immediate cause of death in chronically ill old people; the more so in men than in women due to a higher incidence of chronic bronchitis which inhibits recovery. It is an infection of the alveoli of the lungs which fill with infected exudate and become consolidated.

Lobar pneumonia is caused by a specific micro-organism such as the pneumococcus or a virus, and the infection is usually confined to one lung.

Bronchopneumonia is seen more commonly in elderly people and here the infection is patchy throughout the lungs. *Aspiration pneumonia* may either follow an infection such as influenza or acute bronchitis when the patient has difficulty in coughing and clearing his lungs of secretions, or it may be caused by the inhalation of some foreign matter like food or vomitus, when the swallowing or ejection mechanisms are impaired, as they may be after a stroke. *Hypostatic pneumonia* occurs after a period of immobility, as, for example, when a patient lies helpless for several hours after a fall, or when the patient is confined to bed after an operation. Secretions gather in the lungs and are not coughed up in the normal way because the patient is too weak. It is the particular complication of hypothermia (page 61).

The onset of bronchopneumonia in the elderly, particularly those already immobile or debilitated, can be so rapid that without immediate treatment the patient may lose consciousness and die within a few hours. Alternatively, the onset may be insidious, the patient first appearing unwell and gradually becoming more confused and reluctant to eat and drink. Although her temperature may be sub-normal the pulse and respiration rates will be raised.

The nurse in a geriatric ward should continually be alert to the danger of any patient developing pneumonia and must record and report any changes in the condition of a previously alert patient such as a raised respiratory rate or confused behaviour.

Death from pneumonia is normally peaceful, as the patient is usually unconscious for several hours and is seldom distressed by dyspnoea in the terminal stages. It can, however, occur extremely quickly, particularly at night, and relatives may be very upset at the rapid deterioration in a patient's condition or by her sudden death.

The treatment of a patient with pneumonia. The patient with pneumonia will need the most vigilant care, being nursed in bed sitting upright supported by pillows and backrest, and turned from side to side two-hourly to prevent stasis of the exudate in the lungs and pressure sores from developing. The respiration, pulse rate and temperature should be recorded hourly. The patient must be encouraged to drink, and a check should be kept on her urinary output.

Antibiotic treatment must be started as soon as possible as the onset of pneumonia is so rapid. In severe cases it is usual to give the first few doses by intramuscular injection. Oxygen given at two to three litres per minute will increase the oxygen supply to the brain and calm a restless patient.

As pneumonia is so frequently the immediate cause of death in elderly patients the doctor may make a decision against treatment of the condition in certain patients provided that any associated suffering and pain are controllable. The ethical questions that arise when such a decision is made have become entangled in the euthanasia debate of recent years. In fact the two issues are quite separate as the doctor is not hastening death but is allowing the patient to die peacefully from natural causes. In many cases, even when it has been decided to treat pneumonia, the onset is so rapid and the infection so virulent that the treatment is of no use.

Tuberculosis. It is not yet possible to dismiss pulmonary tuberculosis in this country as a disease of the past, especially in geriatric wards, for here the patients are survivors of an age when it was common and many may have been infected. An infection that has been dormant for many years may become active again particularly if the patient has been living in poor conditions and on an inadequate diet. Unfortunately, because a chronic cough is so common in old age, particularly in old men who smoke, elderly people do not go for routine chest X-rays or seek treatment from the doctor. The disease may only be discovered on admission to hospital for some unrelated cause, by which time it will have been established for years.

While the infection will probably respond to the primary anti-tubercular drugs (Streptomycin, para-aminosalicylic acid (P A S) and isonicotnic acid hydrazide (I N A H) the danger is that by the time treatment is effective the patient may have infected many other people, particularly close relatives, or tenants in a shared house.

4. Diseases of the skeletal system

Osteo-arthritis. Osteo-arthritis is a degenerative condition of the joints caused by wear and tear within the structure of the joint. The joints that take the greatest strain – the hip and knee joints, and the intervertebral joints particularly in the cervical region – are the most likely to be affected especially in obese people, and any joint that has previously been injured is susceptible to arthritic changes. The cartilage within the joint degenerates with age and use, the articulating surfaces are no longer smooth and regular and the space between them is narrowed; the bones making up the joint become hardened, and small overgrowths of bone known as osteophytes develop at the edges of the joint, particularly of the vertebrae.

The joints affected become stiff, swollen and at times very painful. Some patients say the pain is worse in damp weather, others complain of more pain and stiffness after sitting still. As the joints become more deformed, movement is limited and when the hips and knees are affected walking and sitting may be difficult. One of the dangers of decreased mobility is that the patient will not make the effort to move but will sit or lie in one position so that the joints become fixed as the muscles and ligaments contract through disuse. Contractures are difficult to correct and are very disabling as the patient will be unable to stand with a hip or knee joint fixed in a flexed position.

There is no cure for osteo-arthritis but with surgery it is possible to alleviate the symptoms and pain. The hip can be restored with one of a variety of prostheses, or the hip and knee joints can be fixed (arthrodesed) to relive the pain. Medical treatment to retain the mobility of a joint will involve exercising the affected joints and in hospital the physiotherapist can supervise a variety of exercises to improve their functioning (see Chapter 8 – Rehabilitation). Analgesics should be given regularly and a heat lamp or warmed wax treatment can also ease the pain. If the patient is overweight and can be encouraged to diet, the loss of weight will reduce strain on the joints.

Osteo-arthritis is probably the greatest cause of reduced mobility in the elderly and inactivity increases the risk of hypothermia, pneumonia and falls.

Rheumatoid arthritis. The cause of rheumatoid arthritis is not known but it is a condition of generalised inflammation of the joints and comes within the group of Collagen diseases. The onset is usually an acute, self-limiting illness with a raised body temperature, inflamed joints, anaemia and general systemic disturbance. It may occur at any time from middle age onwards and often seems to follow a physical illness or a severe emotional trauma. The periods of acute exacerbation recur and alternate with quiescent periods until the disease is 'burnt out'. Joints particularly affected are the proximal interphalangeal joints, the metacarpal and wrist joints, the elbows, knees, hips and ankles and the feet with a symmetrical distribution. The destruction within the joints is severe, causing gross deformity, so that functionally they may be of little use. Eventually they may become fixed and if the hip and knee joints are involved, walking may no longer be possible. The feet may also become quite misshapen so that it is difficult to get shoes to fit at all and if the joints of the hand and fingers are affected, fine movements, such as those needed to do up buttons, are extremely difficult.

The treatment of the patient with rheumatoid arthritis. Treatment is by drugs aimed at relieving the pain and reducing the inflammation, but unfortunately the best analgesics which are also anti-inflammatory – aspirin and phenylbutazone – can have serious toxic effects if taken over long periods. Both can irritate the gastric mucosa causing chronic bleeding, and phenylbutazone can cause dizziness, rashes and aplastic anaemia. Ibuprofen, a drug specifically for arthritis, is less toxic, but paracetamol, although less toxic is not so effective. Steroids injected into the joints may be used to reduce local inflammation.

If the patient is very anaemic, a blood transfusion can be given, but there is always the danger with elderly patients that extra blood may overload the circulation and precipitate cardiac failure (see page 33).

The nursing care of the patient with rheumatoid arthritis. Nursing care during an acute episode is all-important. The patient must be made as comfortable as possible with the use of a ripple bed and pillows, the weight of the bed clothes being taken by a bed cradle. The patient will be the best judge of how she can be made most comfortable. Splints may be used when the patient is at rest to support the affected joints, which will be extremely painful, and to prevent contractures.

Once the acute inflammation has subsided, heat treatment

from warmed wax or a lamp may be used to ease the joints before giving carefully graded exercises on each occasion. The occupational therapist will be able to supply a variety of aids to help the patient (see Chapter 8).

Although the acute stage of rheumatoid arthritis occurs less frequently in old age, younger patients may be found in geriatric wards because of the chronic nature of the disease. Older patients with long standing rheumatoid arthritis may be admitted for assessment and rehabilitation.

Cervical spondylosis. Many elderly people have arthritic changes of the vertebral column where some of the intervertebral discs have crumbled, causing the vertebra themselves to overlap, and small osteophytes to form at the edge of the bones. Arthritis of the spine is rarely incapacitating although elderly people, once told that they have arthritic changes, will attribute all their backaches to it. Nevertheless, pressure on the sensory and motor nerve pathways leading to or arising from the cervical spine which is affected by arthritis (cervical spondylosis) can cause pain and weakness of the arms and shoulders.

The patient may also suffer from *drop attacks*, when she falls to the ground without warning and without losing consciousness. These attacks occur because the vertebral arteries that run up through the foraminae on either side of the cervical vertebrae to help supply the brain become kinked when the patient's head is twisted suddenly and the blood supply is cut off, causing a temporary ischaemia of the brain.

A lightweight cervical collar may help to relieve the symptoms of pressure on the nerve roots and for the patient who suffers from drop attacks, an explanation of their cause and a warning not to turn the head suddenly may help to prevent further incidents.

Osteoporosis. Osteoporosis is a disease of bones found almost entirely in people over 50 years of age and more commonly in women. The bones become brittle and less dense, probably due to an increased rate of resorbtion of the bone, a decline in dietary calcium and a lack of exercise. One bone only may be affected, especially if it has been immobilised following a fracture, or the condition can be general. The cause of the disease is uncertain but it is an important condition because it can be very crippling. Of great importance to those caring for the elderly is the fact that their long bones are so brittle that they fracture easily, even spontaneously.

In osteoporosis of the spine, when one or more of the vertebrae collapse causing marked kyphosis of the vertebral column, the main symptom is severe backache.

The treatment of the patient with osteoporosis. Despite the pain, increasing kyphosis if the vertebral column is affected, and the risk of fractures, it is important that the patient should remain mobile, for immobility increases the rate of bone resorbtion. Although the bone that remains is normal in structure it is thought that the patient's diet may be deficient in calcium and so extra milk and calcium tablets may be ordered.

The state of the bones may take years to improve but treatment with calcium and anabolic steroids will ease the pain and reduce the risk of fractures. In osteoporosis of the spine, spinal supports or surgical corsets may give some relief, but they are uncomfortable and not well tolerated by elderly people.

5. Anaemia

Anaemia is common in old people but it is not necessarily due to a poor diet. Such is the insidious nature of anaemia, that many old people accept feelings of weakness, lethargy and breathlessness as the effects of age but in fact have been found to have haemoglobin levels as low as 6 g per 100 ml (40 per cent. Haldene). In many cases a patient will be found to be anaemic after being admitted for some other reason, such as cardiac failure, a confusional state or an acute infection.

Iron deficiency anaemia. The body normally stores iron but to maintain an adequate level elderly people need about 10 mg of iron in their daily diet, as iron is being constantly lost from desquamation of the skin and mucus membrane. Unfortunately the foods containing iron – red meat, liver, eggs, green vegetables – are not those which are prominent in the diet of an old person, especially those living alone on a small income. Iron deficiency anaemia due to a poor diet is probably less common than it used to be with the greater availability of meals-on-wheels and luncheon clubs (see Chapter 9) and a growing awareness among people of the need for a balanced diet.

Hydrochloric acid plays a part in the breakdown and absorption of iron; a deficiency of hydrochloric acid (achlorhydria) in the stomach due to atrophy of the stomach lining may be the cause of iron deficiency anaemia, even when there is sufficient iron in the diet (hypochromic, microcytic anaemia).

Chronic bleeding will gradually deplete the body's stores of iron; in old age such bleeding is commonly due to a peptic ulcer, hiatus hernia, diverticulitis or haemorrhoids. Bleeding from the intestinal tract can be detected by an occult blood test of the faeces, and bleeding haemorrhoids will leave streaks of frank blood in the stools. Even if old people know they are losing blood, they may not think it significant enough to do anything about it.

In short, iron deficiency anaemia is due to a low intake, poor absorption or excessive loss of iron.

Treatment of iron deficiency anaemia. The therapy of iron deficiency anaemia is to discover the cause of the deficiency of iron, to treat the cause and to replace the iron. The oral administration of iron, as ferrous sulphate, ferrous glucomate or in other forms, is a slow acting method of replacing iron used when the anaemia is mild and the patient is not achlorhydric. It can however cause nausea, constipation or diarrhoea which may be overcome by changing the iron preparation used.

Intramuscular iron is quick acting but the injections are painful and cause severe bruising. The injections are given daily or on alternate days for about ten doses and are usually followed by a course of oral iron. Intravenous iron may also be given by the doctor, either directly into the vein or in an infusion of saline.

Pernicious anaemia (vitamin B_{12} deficiency anaemia). Pernicious means 'fatal' and until the cause of this form of anaemia was discovered it was indeed fatal. In pernicious anaemia Vitamin B_{12} cannot be absorbed due to the lack of an unidentified substance known as the intrinsic factor, normally present in the gastric juices. Vitamin B_{12} (cyanocobalamine), known as the extrinsic factor, is present in adequate quantities in a well-balanced diet. In some older people (and there is a familial pattern) the stomach lining atrophies and fails to secrete both hydrochloric acid and the intrinsic factor. Vitamin B_{12} is essential for manufacture of healthy red blood cells and if a deficiency is present there will be fewer but large, frail and highly coloured red blood cells produced (hyperchromic, macrocytic anaemia).

The onset of pernicious anaemia is slow as the body has reserves of Vitamin B_{12}. Apart from the usual signs of anaemia – tiredness, pallor, breathlessness and swollen ankles – the patient will have a sore, smooth tongue, lacking papillae, and a characteristic lemon tinge to the skin, due to an early breakdown on the fragile red blood cells and the release of bilirubin.

Lack of Vitamin B_{12} can also cause a peripheral neuritis with numbness and tingling of the feet and hands. Loss of the sensation of pain in the feet, particularly, increases the risk of pressure sores developing without the patient realising it. A more serious neurological effect is the condition known as sub-acute combined degeneration of the spinal cord which will result in permanent damage to the posterior and lateral columns of the cord. This damage will produce a loss of sensory stimuli and cause patients to stumble, particularly in the dark, and to make clumsy, ataxic movements due to a loss of awareness of the position of their limbs in space. The cord damage is progressive and without treatment the patient will become paraplegic. If the deficiency is diagnosed at an early stage and large doses of Vitamin B_{12} are given, the disease will be halted but the neurological damage cannot be reversed.

A form of pernicious anaemia may occur following a partial or total gastrectomy when there will be insufficient intrinsic factor to allow the adequate absorption of Vitamin B_{12}.

Diagnosis and treatment of pernicious anaemia. The diagnosis of pernicious anaemia will be made from a blood film which will show the typical large, fragile cells and from an examination of the bone marrow. A histamine test-meal will also show if acid is being secreted by the stomach; if no acid is present it is unlikely there will be any intrinsic factor either. Treatment is by regular injections of Vitamin B_{12}, at first given daily or on alternate days and then generally reduced to fortnightly or monthly, oral administration of the vitamin being useless. Where there is a neurological involvement the dose of Vitamin B_{12} will be twice that for pernicious anaemia alone. The importance of continuing these injections as prescribed at regular intervals throughout life must be emphasised to the patient before discharge from hospital.

Hypoplasia of the marrow. Another form of anaemia found in the elderly occurs with chronic diseases and appears to be due to a failure of the bone marrow to manufacture sufficient blood cells, which, nevertheless, are normal in colour and in size (normochromic, normocytic anaemia). Anaemia of this type is found in patients with chronic renal failure, where there is long-standing pyelonephritis, rheumatoid arthritis, leukaemia, and other malignant disease including aplastic anaemia, which may follow radiotherapy or radioactive exposure, or treatment with certain drugs.

Anaemia of this type is more difficult to treat, but that occurring with chronic renal failure or rheumatoid arthritis may respond to iron therapy and a well-balanced diet is obviously important. In severe cases a blood transfusion may be necessary.

Care of the elderly patient having a blood transfusion
A blood transfusion may be indicated when a patient has suffered an acute blood loss, such as from a haematemesis, severe haemolysis or hypoplasia, or when there is a need for a rapid rise in the haemoglobin level to aid the healing of large pressure sores. It will only be given when other treatment – parenteral iron or Vitamin B_{12} – will not be effective quickly enough. Severe anaemia can cause hypotension, with the risk of a cerebro-vascular accident, and cardiac or renal failure.

The danger to an elderly patient of a blood transfusion is that the extra volume of fluid may overload the systemic circulation and so precipitate cardiac failure. It is usual to give a packed cell transfusion (in which most of the plasma has been drawn off) so reducing the amount of fluid given; the transfusion must be administered very slowly and a diuretic may be given.

An elderly person undergoing blood transfusion must be carefully observed, have her pulse and respiration rate checked every 15 minutes and her blood pressure and temperature taken hourly. Not only must the nurse watch for signs of a reaction to the transfusion – back pain, rash, possibly a fever or rigor – which may be less dramatic than in a younger patient, but she must also be prepared for the early signs of cardiac failure, atrial fibrillation, breathlessness, confusion and the formation of oedema, particularly in the sacral area.

Following a successful transfusion, the patient's condition improves rapidly. If an old person feels better she will want to eat more and to do more for herself which will be a big step towards her rehabilitation.

6. Endocrine disorders

Diabetes mellitus. Many elderly people have a raised renal threshold for sugar (see Chapter 2) and they may also frequently have a fasting blood sugar level above 120 mg per 100 ml blood which is the normal upper limit for younger adults. As the Clinistix reagent is designed to test the urine of the adult with a normal renal threshold of 160 mg per 100 ml blood it is not a reliable test for older people. A high blood sugar can only be satisfactorily checked by a glucose tolerance test.

An increasing number of lifelong diabetics now reach old age, most of whom will have relied on regular injections of insulin. A less severe form of diabetes occurs in elderly people and appears to be due to an intolerance of insulin or a failure of the Islets of Langerhans in the pancreas to manufacture adequate amounts of insulin. Obesity seems to be an important factor in diabetes of late onset, for many elderly people who are found to be diabetic are overweight, which in some way may increase their insulin intolerance.

The symptoms of diabetes of late onset are usually mild and the condition may only be discovered when the patient is being examined for something else. Polyuria, which will aggravate incontinence (see page 65), thirst, pruritis and lethargy are all symptoms of diabetes which could be dismissed by the patient as being insignificant. The elderly patient is unlikely to go into a hyperglycaemic coma but she may be confused.

Diabetes mellitus may only be discovered as the result of one of its complications. Diabetic patients are prone to develop atherosclerosis, especially of the coronary arteries and the arteries of the lower limbs. Poor circulation in the legs can lead to the development of gangrene and varicose ulcers; and so diabetics must be warned to take particular care of the smallest cut or sore on their legs or feet as it will quickly become infected and be slow to heal. Foot care should be undertaken only by a chiropodist.

Neurological changes occur which cause numbness and tingling in the feet and cramp and pain in the calves, severe enough to cause foot drop. Elderly diabetics frequently develop cataracts and specific changes in the retina which lead to a partial blindness (diabetic retinopathy).

The treatment of a patient with diabetes mellitus. Diabetes of late onset usually occurs in a mild form and may be controlled by limiting the amount of carbohydrate in the patient's diet and by the oral anti-diabetic drugs, such as tolbutamide or chlorpropamide, which stimulate the production of insulin.

Elderly people find it difficult to appreciate the importance of keeping to a diet and as many of them are accustomed to living on the cheaper, carbohydrate foods such as bread, jam, biscuits and potatoes, there may be economic difficulties in changing their diet. It is unlikely that the elderly people will manage to keep to a strict diet in which all food is carefully weighed, and it is usually sufficient to make a list of those foods which should not be eaten – cakes, sweets, chocolate, biscuits and puddings – those which can be eaten in small quantities – bread, potatoes and cereals – and those which can be eaten at will – fruit, vegetables, meat, eggs and fish. The treatment can be effective and the diabetes controlled for those patients who have a relative or neighbour to help them with the shopping, and who will stress the need to continue the diet once they have left hospital. For those patients who live alone, it may be necessary for them to attend a day hospital where for part of the day their diet can be supervised.

In elderly patients, the diabetes is usually so stabilised that there is a small amount of sugar in the urine, enough to lessen the risk of their becoming hypoglycaemic should they eat less than their normal diet on one day. Once the diabetes is controlled, the lethargy, the polyuria and thirst should disappear and the patients' health improve generally. They should, however, be seen regularly at the outpatients' clinic to check that the diabetes is still under control and to reinforce the need for the diet. Even mild diabetic patients are at risk of developing the complications associated with the disease and regular checks will ensure the rapid treatment of these to prevent further handicaps.

Myxoedema or hypothyroidism is a fairly common condition in old age, particularly among women. While it is usually due to a failure of the thyroid gland to secrete thyroxine it may follow a thyroidectomy or excessive treatment of thyrotoxicosis. The symptoms are easily mistaken for those of normal ageing, especially as the onset is very gradual over several years. The most striking changes are a puffiness of the face, especially around the eyes, and a deepening and hoarseness of the voice. Speech too may become slow and indistinct. Other signs are a cold, dry, pale skin; thin brittle hair, tingling of the hands and oversensitivity to cold. These patients' movements are slow and clumsy, their reactions are slow and they may be mildly confused and often constipated.

Patients with myxoedema are often anaemic and may suffer from ischaemic heart disease, although the radial pulse will be slow. As all the body processes function more slowly than is normal, these patients are particularly at risk of becoming hypothermic.

Diagnosis and treatment. The diagnosis of myxoedema is made by blood tests carried out to estimate the amount of circulating thyroid hormone.

The treatment is to give thyroxine orally, starting with a small dose daily, which is increased gradually to a maintenance dose. The patient must continue to take this for the rest of her life. Once treatment has begun, there will be a striking improvement in the patient's reaction, appearance and mental alertness.

Thyrotoxicosis. Thyrotoxicosis or hyperthyroidism can occur in old age and is significant as a cause of cardiac failure because the cardiac output is insufficient to cope with the raised metabolic rate. The patient is likely to be thin, restless and anxious but may not have the usual signs of the condition – exophthalmos and an increased appetite, and the tremor may be mistaken for a senile tremor. Her sleeping pulse will usually be above 80 beats a minute with atrial fibrillation present.

The treatment of the patient with thyrotoxicosis. The most serious complication of thyrotoxicosis in the elderly is heart failure. The patient will be prescribed digoxin to control the atrial fibrillation and an anti-thyroid drug, such as carbimazole or radio-iodine to decrease the activity of the gland, the dosage being reviewed regularly. A partial thyroidectomy may be undertaken in some cases if there is inadequate response to conservative treatment.

SECTION 2. MENTAL DISORDERS OF THE ELDERLY

Many of the elderly people admitted to a geriatric department, whether to the psychogeriatric unit or to the general assessment ward, will show signs of mental disorder. One of the problems faced by a nurse new to geriatric care is understanding the terms – confusion, dementia, senility and so on – used to describe the mental state of elderly people. The tendency of lay people to lump into a general category of 'senility' all types of mental disorder found in the elderly must be resisted, and in order to help to clarify the causes and manifestations of some of the more common disorders these are described briefly.

Another problem in defining mental disorder in this age group is the lack of a clear distinction between changes in the mind and personality due to normal ageing and the changes that occur as a result of an affective or organic disease. The point at which an old person's failing memory and increasing conservatism requires medical treatment may depend largely on the social situation. Kind relatives will tolerate the failing memory of an amiable old person for longer than a landlady will put up with an aggressive lodger whose forgetfulness has led to his leaving the gas on. Impairment of the special senses –

deafness and blindness – may make an old person become withdrawn and even paranoid. There is probably a large number of elderly people with mental disorders who are still able to live in the community without medical attention because they have someone to care for them.

Yet another problem is that sometimes the signs of different mental disorders are similar but the cause may be very different and it is most important to distinguish those conditions which are treatable, particularly acute toxic confusional states, from those conditions in which deterioration is inevitable, as is senile dementia. While the diagnosis is the doctor's responsibility, the nurse's observations of the patient's behaviour can help establish the diagnosis and her own attitude to the patient.

Temporary acute toxic confusional states. Old people who suddenly become confused, disorientated, aggressive, delirious, even hallucinated may be suffering from a physical condition which has upset their mental integrity either by reducing the oxygen supply to the brain or by releasing a toxic substance which affects the precarious balance between the body's systems. It has already been stressed that a confusional state, usually temporary, may be an early sign of many diseases, the sudden, acute onset rather than the degree of the confusion being important. Conditions that may lead to acute toxic confusional states are:

(i) any disease which deprives the brain of oxygen, e g acute bronchitis, cardiac failure, anaemia, hypotension and shock, hypothermia and transient ischaemic attacks;

(ii) other toxic conditions, e g uraemia, dehydration, any acute infection such as sepsis or pneumonia, gangrene thyrotoxicosis, or constipation;

(iii) post-operative states, especially after general anaesthesia;

(iv) the effect of some drugs, e g hypotensive drugs, digoxin, barbiturates, anti-Parkinson drugs and tranquillisers; and

(v) environmental changes such as moving house or admission to hospital, or an emotional shock such as the death of a close relative or friend.

A sudden change in the behaviour of an aged parent can be very distressing for relatives, as the old person who is severely confused can be noisy, violent and abusive. Apart from the immediate problems of controlling the old person, relatives are likely to fear that this is the start of madness which will mean that the old person will have to be sent away to a mental hospital. The stigma of mental illness is still very real and it is considered by some lay people to reflect upon the sanity of other members of the family.

Once the physical condition has been diagnosed and treatment started, the old person's mental state will improve and it is possible that she will have been aware of behaving abnormally and may even be able to give an account of her delusions. The confusion is likely to recur with any acute illness.
Dementia. Dementia is an intellectual impairment which occurs as the result of organic changes in the brain. There are considered to be two causes of dementia.

(*i*) *Senile dementia.* Physical changes in the brain of patients with senile dementia show atrophy of the brain cells with widening of the sulci and degenerative changes in the nerve cells. More women suffer than men from this form of dementia and there may be a genetic factor in the incidence of this condition.

True senile dementia is a gradual and continuous process of deterioration of the old person's intellect and in the later stages, a disintegration of the personality. At first such patients may be muddled and forgetful but after a time their speech will become confused and repetitive; they may be disorientated, wander at night and suffer from paranoid delusions. As their personality disintegrates they will neglect personal hygiene and appearance and become insensitive to other people's feelings. At this stage such patients are usually no longer able to be cared for in the community and they will have to be admitted to hospital for long-term care where they will eventually die of a degenerative disease or an acute infection.

(*ii*) *Cerebral arteriosclerotic dementia.* In this form of dementia, changes in the brain are the result of ischaemic episodes that leave small, widespread infarcted areas which will gradually destroy the intellect. These episodes are more in the nature of transient ischaemic attacks (see page 26) than a full stroke, but the mental impairment will be similar to that which may follow a stroke. Parkinsonism and hypertension are commonly present and the condition occurs more frequently in men. While the intellect deteriorates and the emotions are labile, the basic personality does not deteriorate as it does in senile dementia and so the patient may remain quite amiable. The progress of the disease is not continuous and on some days it may partly regress so that the patient appears to behave quite normally. The patient will usually die of a severe cerebro-vascular accident.

There is no really effective treatment for either form of dementia and the patient may suffer from a mixture of the two types. In its early stages the old person may be able to live at home in familiar surroundings with a well ordered routine. As the patient's condition deteriorates, more supervised care will usually be necessary.

Affective disorders. An affective disorder is a condition in which there is a serious disturbance of mood.

(i) *Depression.* It has been estimated that as many as one quarter of people over 65 years of age in this country suffer from depression but the symptoms are frequently unrecognised and may be put down to old age.

Reactive depression. Old people have to contend with many personal changes and events which even the most extrovert must find depressing. Mobility is restricted and loss of sight and hearing can have a devastating effect and make future independence uncertain. A small income makes the cost of living a constant worry and when contemporaries die leaving them increasingly isolated and lonely, conditions become intolerable. It would be unnatural if, in such circumstances, old people did not sometimes have feelings of misery, grief, apathy and depression. Yet given the support of understanding friends and relatives, or in some cases the help of the statutory services (see Chapter 9), most old people will overcome depression which is a reaction to a particular event without resort to medical help; in some cases, the depression is triggered off by a distressing episode and is more than a normal reaction, or the old person is so isolated that the help the support is not there when it is needed and the depression overwhelms her.

Endogenous depression. Endogenous depression is a psychotic illness which may be precipitated by an emotional crisis but the depression that results is more deep seated and does not pass as circumstances improve. These patients are likely to have suffered previously from depression or anxiety.

An early sign of depression in old people is an unreasonable concern for their own health (hypochondria) and they complain of minor aches and pains, palpitations, constipation and fears that they may have a serious illness. Anxiety commonly occurs with depression, so that at times the old person may be restless, agitated and have paranoid delusions.

As this type of depression deepens, old people become more apathetic and neglectful, withdrawing into themselves and answering questions only in monosyllables. In an extreme state they may sit, huddled in a chair, incontinent and refusing to eat. Periods of lethargy may alternate with periods of agitation when they will wander round the house at night and even go outside in a distressed state. Suicide attempts are not uncommon. It is this behaviour that alarms neighbours into sending for the doctor and which can give a misleading impression of dementia.

The intellect of the depressed person is not impaired, as it is with true dementia, so that with patience and understanding the patient may be persuaded to answer questions rationally. The observant nurse may notice signs of a normal response to questions and this must be recorded and reported to the doctor.

Treatment. If depression is diagnosed early, elderly people can recover and return home after treatment with antidepressant drugs such as amitriptyline and imipramine, or the doctor may occasionally recommend electro-convulsive therapy. Such patients may be able to attend a psychogeriatric day hospital or they may benefit from mixing with patients in the geriatric day hospital.

Managing the depressed patient in the ward is discussed in Chapter 6.

Late paraphrenia. Late paraphrenia is a mental disorder of the elderly and is thought to be a form of schizophrenia. It takes the form of severe delusions which colour or even control the patient's behaviour and way of life. Typically, the old people live alone, are very isolated, have probably led an upright, restricted life and may be partially deaf or blind.

Such patients feel that someone – a neighbour, the police or an unknown agent – is spying on them by using electricity, radio waves or a special ray gun and is trying to destroy them. The delusions, which are often sexual in nature, may be so severe as to prevent patients from going outside and they may cover all their windows. They will offer apparently rational explanations for their behaviour but may have sufficient insight into their condition as to be willing to accept help from a doctor. On the other hand, relatives or neighbours may seek medical help when such patients are obviously neglecting themselves.

Treatment. Treatment with tranquillising drugs or electro-convulsive therapy is rarely effective and these old people may have to be admitted into residential care. Provided their delusions are reasonably tolerated, they should be able to care for themselves and be acceptable patients in a home for the mentally infirm rather than being admitted to the long-stay ward of a geriatric or psychiatric hospital.

SECTION 3. THE HAZARDS OF OLD AGE

When a nurse has worked for a short time in the assessment ward of a geriatric department she will realise that some patients are there for other than solely medical reasons. Certain conditions – hypothermia, incontinence – are symptomatic of a social as much as a medical breakdown and a situation arises when an old person can no longer live independently and, rightly or wrongly, is admitted to hospital.

1. Social breakdown

Failure of support. It is a sad fact that some elderly people, particularly those who live alone, have such a tenuous hold on their independence that failure of the support from a relative or neighbour upon whom they have come to rely may lead to a crisis that results in their being admitted to hospital. Most elderly people need some help with shopping, housework and the heavier chores and some require help with washing, cooking and bathing. If this help ceases they will be unable to manage. Elderly people depend on an established routine and may resent a neighbour helping out while a daughter is on holiday, or may become too dependent upon a friend, who then moves away from the area. In some cases a home help or home nurse can provide the service needed but it may be that the relative or neighbour has provided not only the support but an essential relationship in the old person's life which cannot instantly be met by someone else.

The rationale of admitting such people to hospital is questionable. The more appropriate move to sheltered housing or a local authority old people's home may just not be possible immediately (see Chapter 9). Very often it is some crisis such as a fall (see page 65) or a burn that brings old people who are struggling to manage alone to the casualty department of their district hospital, later to be admitted to the geriatric department. In this respect a geriatric ward serves a protective function not found in other parts of the hospital (except perhaps in the paediatric ward where a child is admitted to protect it from parental abuse). Such patients are not strictly in need of medical care and there is a danger of their becoming too dependent in hospital. They need to re-establish their independence and the place for this is not in hospital but in the community.

Some geriatric departments will admit elderly people while relatives or friends who supply the essential support are away on holiday; other units may operate a rotation system of three months in, three months out, for patients who are totally dependent upon the support of a relative, without whose care they would be hospitalised anyway. Support is maintained by the hospital for a limited period to allow the relative respite from the arduous task of caring for the old person.

Loss of confidence. Some elderly people live quite competently at home until a crisis occurs and their whole existence begins to fall apart.

Bereavement. The death of a partner or close companion can precipitate a crisis even if the one who survives has been the stronger partner. The old person is suddenly left alone, ill-prepared for the death of the person upon whom their own life has in some way depended. Their purpose in life has gone. Even where relatives step in to help, the shock and sense of loss can leave the old person without confidence or a desire to live and it is not uncommon for husband and wife to die within a few weeks of each other.

Illness. Any minor illness or accident can be a crisis which results in loss of confidence. A short spell in bed, which means a change of routine, can leave old people apathetic and fearful of having to cope again. A fall, particularly if old people have had to lie on the floor for a long time before help comes, may cause such lack of confidence that they become chairbound.

Change of routine. A change in routine, such as a move, taking a holiday or even a spell of bad weather that keeps the old people from going to their club, can be the precipitating factor that brings about loss of confidence.

The onset of social breakdown brought about by a loss of confidence is not usually a sudden occurrence but an insidious process, apparent perhaps to neighbours and friends but not always to the old people themselves, who begin to show signs of anxiety and inability to cope with everyday tasks. They may be frightened to go out and can become depressed (see page 56). Old people in this situation may struggle on for some time before falling ill with an infection, or even hypothermia, which will require medical care in hospital, where their problems will be assessed and help provided. Rehabilitation will be important if the patients are to have their confidence restored and their independence regained. It could be argued that cases of social breakdown would be better treated within the community from which the problems arise rather than by taking the old people away from the environment they know to an institution upon which they may become too dependent. It is essential to look at the needs of the patient as a whole, and not their physical, mental or social problems or needs in isolation.

A case history illustrates how an old person may come to be admitted to hospital:

'Mrs F., a widow for many years, had extensive osteo-arthritis but managed to care for herself in her small, well-equipped flat. She was, however, dependent upon her daughter living nearby for all her shopping, heavy housework and help with her bath. When her daughter's husband was admitted to hospital with a severe heart attack, her daughter was no longer able to visit her so often. Despite the efforts of a home help and home nurse to fill the gap, Mrs F. resented the interference of strangers, and struggled on with a neighbour doing her shopping, becoming more discontented and intolerant despite the many attempts to help. It seems that her daughter has not only provided the physical help but has been an essential source of companionship in Mrs F's restricted life. Over a period of a few weeks Mrs F. had several falls and after one incident, when she lay helpless for several hours, her doctor requested a home visit by the geriatrician. It was arranged that Mrs F. should be admitted to hospital for a short period of rehabilitation by which time her daughter would be able to spend more time with her, and to follow this with a twice-weekly attendance at the geriatric day hospital. Although Mrs F. was still physically able to continue to live at home, she had lost her confidence and for a time the essential support from her daughter. The day hospital would give Mrs F. a chance to meet other people and make her less reliant upon her daughter for social contact.'

2. Hypothermia

Hypothermia is a condition that has attracted much attention in both medical and lay circles in the last few years. It is a condition in which the deep body temperature falls below 35°C (95°F) due to a failure of the temperature regulating mechanism; it is an extremely dangerous state and frequently results in death. Most cases occur in winter, particularly in the late winter months (February and March) but the condition can occur in cool, summer periods. Prevention of hypothermia is the most important aspect of the condition and for this it is necessary to understand the causes.

Hypothermia following an accident occurs as the result of exposure. The elderly person falls, perhaps while getting out of bed at night and may lie for several hours on the floor, inadequately covered in a cold room so that body heat is lost. Shock and pain from an injury sustained in the fall will lower the blood pressure and so reduce the body temperature still further.

All elderly people living alone are open to the risk of falling and lying for some time before help comes. The number of these incidents can be reduced by making sure that old people have sufficient aids to help them move about easily and that the passageways and stairs in the house are well lit and free from obstructions, torn carpets and trailing wires. Adequate room heating is essential to help the body maintain its temperature should the old person lie helpless on the floor. Heating is extremely expensive for the pensioner living on a small income and many elderly people used to sleeping in unheated rooms will be unwilling to spend extra money on heating, especially in their bedrooms. Hypothermia following a fall may be prevented by an effective alarm system, particularly of the type which is fitted to the lavatory flushing system and will ring if the lavatory has not been flushed for more than eight hours, and by the constant vigilance of neighbours and tradespeople.
Hypothermia of insidious onset. While hypothermia following an accident should be easily recognised, it can occur also in elderly people who show few signs of illness. Lowering of the body temperature may be the result of a pathological condition such as myxoedema, a cerebro-vascular accident or the effects of some drugs, particularly chlorpromazine, which affects the temperature regulating centre. Apart from recognisable causes, general immobility, malnutrition and neglect as the result of mental disorder may, over a period, lead to a lowering of body temperature of which the elderly people are unaware. Old people with hypothermia are commonly thought to live in squalid isolation, neglecting themselves, but they can also become hypothermic in a centrally-heated flat, particularly if they are chairbound or can move only with difficulty. Any chairbound patients in a hospital ward are also at risk, particularly where there are fluctuating weather conditions, when the level of the ward heating may have been reduced.

The onset of hypothermia occurring over several days may

accompany an acute infection such as bronchitis, a mild cerebro-vascular accident or a coronary thrombosis when the blood pressure is low. At first the old person will be apathetic or mildly confused, with slow, slurred speech, but as the temperature falls will become comatose. The old person will appear pale, with ruddy, flushed cheeks and oedematous face. The respirations will be slow and shallow, blood pressure low and the muscles in spasm. Above all, the skin of the abdomen and thighs, despite their being covered, will feel cold and clammy and when the temperature is below 32°C (about 90°F) there will be no shivering, the normal reaction of skeletal muscles to contract in an attempt to maintain body temperature. A low temperature, taken rectally, will confirm the diagnosis.

Many of the signs listed above are vague enough to be missed by a relative or visiting neighbour, particularly if there is nothing else to suggest that the patient is ill, and this is where the danger lies. To prevent this tragic condition all who care for the elderly, whether from the statutory services, voluntary services or relatives and neighbours, must be taught to recognise the old people who are at risk and the signs that might indicate the onset of hypothermia. Prevention must include the encouragement of elderly people to be mobile, to wear adequate, suitable clothing, to use more heating and to eat a mixed diet with plenty of hot drinks.

The treatment of patients with hypothermia. Any patients with a rectal temperature below 35°C are dangerously ill and should be admitted to hospital. Ideally, any patients found to have even mild hypothermia are best treated in hospital unless their home circumstances are good, there is adequate heating and someone willing to care for them.

The most important part of the treatment is to warm patients SLOWLY at the rate of about $\frac{1}{2}$°C an hour. While it is a great temptation to surround them with hot water bottles, overheating will cause dilatation of the capillaries which will lower the blood pressure even further and cause a total collapse. To warm a patient up slowly she must be placed in bed with several loose blankets, in a room temperature of at least 24°C (75°F). During the process the rectal temperature, pulse and blood pressure must be taken hourly to ensure that the patient is not getting warm too quickly. As an old person is likely to be dehydrated, if conscious and able to accept them, warm drinks should be given frequently, but if the patient is unable to drink, an intravenous infusion may be started by the doctor. Hydrocortisone may be ordered and given intravenously to help restore the blood pressure. The serious complication of hypothermia is bronchopneumonia for which the doctor may prescribe a prophylactic course of antibiotics.

Despite the greatest care some patients appear to recover but then relapse and die a few days after admission. It is hoped that with the growing concern about the living conditions of old people and awareness of the dangers of hypothermia, it will be prevented, or should hypothermia occur it will be recognised early, when treatment can be very effective.

3. Accidents and falls

Old people are particularly prone to accidents both in the home and out in the street. Their movements and reactions are slower, including the ability to regain balance; their eyesight, hearing and sense of smell less perceptive and their concentration less acute. As well as these effects of ageing, many will suffer from diseases which will affect their balance or cause them to faint or collapse without warning.

The effect of the accident may be out of all proportion to what has occurred. Old people's bones fracture easily and a fractured femur may mean an operation and months of rehabilitation. Even when there is no fracture, a fall may cause the old person to lose confidence and become unable to manage without help. The shock of an accident may precipitate a temporary confusional state necessitating admission to hospital and a period of rehabilitation to help the old person to regain confidence.

The prevention of accidents in the home. Once it is recognised that old people are more prone to accidents than younger people, their home environment can be adapted, usually quite easily, to help prevent them.

Accidental falls can be avoided by removing slip mats from highly polished floors, fixing stair-carpet rods, putting up extra banisters and eliminating such hazards as trailing flexes, poorly lit stairs and passageways. Burns and scalds can be prevented by using fireguards, safety paraffin heaters and mixer taps on baths and kitchen sinks. Good lighting in the kitchen will help to prevent many small accidents, like burns and cuts from utensils, which for an old person may mean the loss of independence if unable to manage alone with a bandaged hand.

Coal gas poisoning is no longer a great problem as most houses use natural gas, but there is always the risk of explosion if the gas is accidentally left on or of poisoning from the effect of inefficient appliances in poorly ventilated rooms. Old people may need to be encouraged to have their gas appliances serviced regularly. Accidental poisoning from drugs is always a risk among the elderly who usually have a large number of prescribed and patent medicines around the house and who may not be able to read the labels or remember for which condition they were prescribed. Old people must be persuaded to throw away unused medicine and tablets.

The prevention of accidents in the street. Old people and the very young are the groups most likely to be involved in traffic accidents. Shopping precincts in towns, pedestrian controlled crossings that allow an old person time to get across the road and a greater awareness and consideration on the part of drivers, will all help to reduce accidents. The elderly can be reminded of the dangers of traffic and the best ways to cross the road through talks to old people's clubs by health visitors or others who care for the aged. Falls that occur in the street are often due to uneven pavements; as old people tend not to lift up their feet they risk tripping over loose paving stones, unexpected steps and other small hazards.

Prevention does not mean confining the old person to bed or a chair, in order to prevent the chance of an accident. Many old people realise that they are at greater risk of falling and will carry a stick or move around more cautiously. Some will state that they prefer to live independently and risk having an accident than live under constant supervision in an old people's home.

Falls. Falls account for the largest number of accidents suffered by old people and are responsible for serious injury and death. Old people are liable to accidental falls but some falls can partly be due to the effects of an existing physical disturbance. Many old people suffer from giddiness or vertigo which may be due to degenerative changes in the inner ear affecting the balance mechanism (Ménière's Disease), postural hypotension or the effect of some drugs, but in many cases the cause is not known. Drop attacks (page 44) account for some of the falls of old people. Conditions which cause a temporary hypoxia of the brain, like Stokes-Adams' attacks (page 33), transient ischaemic attacks (page 26) and myocardial infarctions may cause old people to collapse and even lose consciousness. In the home there is a danger they may fall either onto a fire or downstairs, causing far more serious injuries than the episode warrants.

Accidents in the ward are discussed in Chapter 7.

4. Incontinence of urine

Some patients will be in a geriatric ward principally because they are incontinent. There comes a point when relatives and neighbours will no longer cope with the extra washing and unpleasant smell that occurs with persistent incontinence when the old person is dependent upon them for support. Yet in the majority of cases the cause of the incontinence is not pathological but accidental, arising from inadequate facilities or insufficient help and the need is for social support rather than medical care.

Accidental incontinence. In old age, slackening of the connective tissue supporting the bladder and weakening of the pelvic floor muscles will cause the bladder to become funnel-shaped and will impair the efficiency of the sphincter. As the bladder capacity also decreases with age and the muscular walls become increasingly irritable, frequency and precipitancy are more likely to occur. In normal circumstances, this should cause no special problem but if some reason – illness, immobility, or distance – makes it difficult for the old person to reach the lavatory, the combination of frequency, precipitancy and an inefficient sphincter will result in lack of continence. Similarly, the old person who relies upon help to get to the lavatory will lack continence if the assistance is delayed.

When incontinence first occurs in an old person who hitherto has had no problem, it is usually possible to point to some incident that has precipitated it; perhaps an illness, a urinary infection, a fall that has left the old person unsteady, an emotional upset or a move. Accidental incontinence may be aggravated by depression or tension within the family.

Many cases of accidental incontinence will improve as the situation which precipitated them resolves. If the problem is, for instance, an old lady whose arthritis is so severe in damp weather that she cannot get to the lavatory quickly enough because it is down a flight of stairs but can manage if she has a commode, there should be no need for the intervention of the geriatrician. However, when the cause is not obvious, or when it is tied up with other issues, like an old lady's difficult personality or the relatives' reluctance to continue supporting her, incontinence may be used as an excuse for her to be admitted to hospital, which will not solve the problems that have led to her incontinence. Hospitalisation may in fact increase the nocturnal incontinence because the patient does not want to disturb the ward by getting up, or is discouraged from doing so by the nursing staff, who at the same time may be slow to bring a bedpan or commode when asked. It is regrettable that nocturnal incontinence is still accepted as almost inevitable in some hospital wards.

The apathy and weakness of old people which can prevent them from reaching the lavatory may have a medical cause, such as anaemia, myxoedema or depression and which will need treatment, although not necessarily in hospital. There is a danger that accidental incontinence will become habitual if the true reason for it is not discovered and relieved. This is most likely to occur in the long-stay wards of hospitals where it is too easy to accept incontinence, where sedative drugs, perhaps, are given out too readily or where there are insufficient staff to attend to the patients. The management of incontinence is discussed in Chapter 7.

Pathological causes. Incontinence in some patients is due to a pathological condition which affects voluntary control of the bladder or damages the bladder or surrounding organs.

Bladder control. The bladder is under the control of the parasympathetic division of the autonomic nervous system arising from branches of the second, third and fourth sacral nerves on either side of the spinal cord. After the spinal cord receives afferent impulses from the bladder indicating that its normal capacity has been reached, efferent motor impulses are transmitted from the anterior horn cells of the cord to the muscles of the bladder wall, causing them to contract, and to the external urethral sphincter, causing it to relax and open the exit. The act of micturition can be inhibited by higher voluntary control from the cerebral cortex which will only allow the external sphincter to be relaxed at an appropriate time.

Loss of bladder control. Damage to the higher control as the result of a cerebro-vascular accident or temporary ischaemia of the brain results in the bladder contracting strongly when only partially filled, causing frequency and precipitancy. Where cerebral damage has caused dementia, the patient may not have the motivation to control her micturition and in extreme cases all cerebral control is lost and the reflex control takes over, as in a baby.

Local damage and infection. (i) *Stress incontinence* occurs in women when the pelvic floor muscles have become lax, usually following childbirth. The prolapsed uterus will distort the angle between the neck of the bladder and the urethra and any sudden increase in intra-abdominal pressure, such as a cough or a laugh, will force a little urine through the incompetent sphincter. Women may be reluctant to go to their doctor for advice, although they are conscious of pelvic discomfort, and they may have to wear a pad to cope with the stress incontinence. These patients are particularly at risk of infection ascending the bladder.

Treatment of this form of stress incontinence is by repair surgery to tighten the muscles of the pelvic floor and the ligaments supporting the uterine cervix, which is a relatively minor operation suitable for older patients. For very elderly women, or those not suitable for general anaesthesia, a ring pessary can be inserted into the vagina which will support the uterus and correct the angle between the bladder neck and the uterus.

(ii) *Retention of urine with overflow* is more common among older male patients, when a benign (or occasionally malignant) enlargement of the prostate gland constricts the neck of the bladder. The patient will complain of a constant dribbling of urine, which may be mistaken for true incontinence. A distended bladder may be palpable above the symphysis pubis and the patient will have pain on micturition and haematuria. Chronic distension of the bladder can lead to urinary infection due to stagnation of urine, and to pressure on the kidneys causing renal damage.

Treatment of an enlarged prostate is by prostatectomy, either retro-pubic or through the urethra via a cystoscope (trans-urethral), which can be carried out successfully despite the patient's age, but where physical or mental health is poor it may be more suitable to insert an indwelling catheter. If it is necessary to pass a catheter to empty a chronically distended bladder, the urine must be drained slowly over several hours to prevent sudden decompression which may cause shock and bleeding from the kidneys. Catheter care is discussed more fully in Chapter 7.

A rectum full of hard faeces, a stricture of the bladder neck, or bladder stones, any of which exerts pressure on the urethra or bladder neck can be the cause of retention of urine with overflow.

(iii) Infection. A urinary infection is frequently a contributory cause of accidental incontinence because it increases the irritability of the bladder. Infection is common in elderly women particularly where there has been some disturbance of micturition, such as following a stroke, or in stress incontinence. Women whose personal hygiene is poor or whose facilities for washing are inadequate and who are unable to keep the perineal area clean are particularly at risk of infection in the bladder (cystitis). If the vulva is contaminated by diarrhoea it must be cleansed immediately to prevent the risk of cystitis occurring. The *Esterichia coli* (E. coli) organisms which are commensals (non-pathogenic) in their normal habitat in the large bowel, become highly pathogenic in the urinary tract and are the commonest cause of urinary infection. However, urinary infections of unknown aetiology are very common.

The infecting organism will need to be identified, if possible, from a mid-stream specimen of urine before specific treatment with antibiotics, chemotherapeutic agents or urinary antiseptics can be effective. Infection is likely to recur and it is helpful to try to identify the cause.

5. Constipation

Constipation is common in elderly people, particularly those who are relatively inactive and whose diet is poor. Nurses tend to make light of an elderly person's complaint of constipation but it can be a very distressing condition, causing anxiety, restlessness, temporary acute toxic confusional states, anorexia, and incontinence of urine. While constipation may be symptomatic of diverticulitis, haemorrhoids or a tumour of the lower bowel, in the main it is due to a combination of poor diet with too little roughage and fluids, an inadequate or inaccessible lavatory and a life-long habit of taking aperients.

Constipation is not usually the primary cause of a patient's admission to hospital; an old person who is very constipated may in fact complain of diarrhoea. Faecal incontinence is the least socially acceptable condition and will quickly lead to a breakdown in the support an old person is receiving.

Rectal dyschezia. The normal stimulus to defaecate is the sensation of a full rectum but in old age this sensation may be diminished causing the rectum to become full of hard, impacted faeces, the condition known as dyschezia. If the mass of faeces in the rectum prevents the anal sphincter from closing, faecal matter may leak from higher up the bowel causing spurious diarrhoea. Such a patient may make her constipation worse by taking kaolin to prevent the diarrhoea.

Treatment. The removal of hard, impacted faeces, which may occur with or without spurious diarrhoea, is likely to take several days. When the rectum is full of hard faeces, aperients are usually ineffective and may cause painful spasms of the bowel. Suppositories may be sufficient to clear the rectum but it is probable that an olive oil or a glycerine enema which is retained for several hours will be needed to soften the faeces, followed by an evacuant enema to clear the bowel. This treatment may have to be repeated once or twice until the rectum and sigmoid colon is quite clear.

A bowel which has been grossly distended with faeces will

lack muscle tone and to prevent it becoming impacted again it may be necessary to give the patient an enema or suppositories regularly once a week. For a patient who is immobile, a regular enema given in conjunction with an agent to keep the faeces soft, such as Dioctyl, might be the least traumatic way of ensuring a regular emptying of the bowel.

A manual evacuation of hard, impacted faeces should be undertaken only with the consent of the doctor. It is a painful and distressing procedure for the patient and carries the risk that the bowel may be perforated if there are diverticulae present.

Prevention. Constipation in the elderly can be prevented without giving regular aperients, by encouraging old people to alter their dietary habits. If they could be encouraged to drink more fluids, especially a hot drink first thing in the morning, and to take two tablespoons of bran cereal daily, they should have regular, soft bowel motions. However, lifelong habits and attitudes are difficult to change.

Improving lavatory conditions is a far more difficult problem but an elderly person may find life easier if a commode is placed beside her bed.

For Further Reading

Agate, J. *The Practice of Geriatrics.* Heinemann, 1970

Bromley, D. B. *The Psychology of Human Ageing.* Penguin Books, 1966

Laurence, D. R. *Clinical Pharmacology.* Churchill-Livingstone, 1976

Thompson, M. K. *Geriatrics and the General Practitioner Team.* Baillière, Tindall, 1969

Whitehead, J. A. *Psychiatric Disorders in Old Age.* H M + M Publishers, 1974

5. The Geriatric Department

As the specialty of geriatric medicine has developed over the last 25 years, so the geriatric department has evolved. Although hospitals throughout the country have developed their own facilities for treating the elderly to suit local needs, a common approach is emerging, based upon three principles.

Firstly, elderly patients can be treated effectively. After rehabilitation they can return to their own homes and do not necessarily have to become long-stay patients as they would have done 30 years ago. Secondly, the concept of progressive care has come about because it has been realised that each stage in an old person's treatment needs a different approach and different equipment. The aim is to make full use of the resources available and to treat the patient in the best possible environment, by moving her to the most suitable place for her care. Thirdly, the importance of community care has been realised so that geriatric departments extend their care beyond the hospital and with day hospitals actually help to co-ordinate home and hospital care. Figure 1 shows in diagrammatic form the arrangement of a typical geriatric department and how a patient may progress through it.

Admission

An elderly person is usually referred to the geriatric physician by her general practitioner. The physician may arrange to see the patient either in the outpatients' clinic or in her own home. The advantage of a home visit is that the doctor meets the patient and the relatives on their own ground where they can talk more freely of their hopes and anxieties; he can assess the patient's background, her need for rehabilitation and for domiciliary services on returning home. The patient may more readily accept admission (and many elderly people strongly resist the idea of going into hospital) if she has already

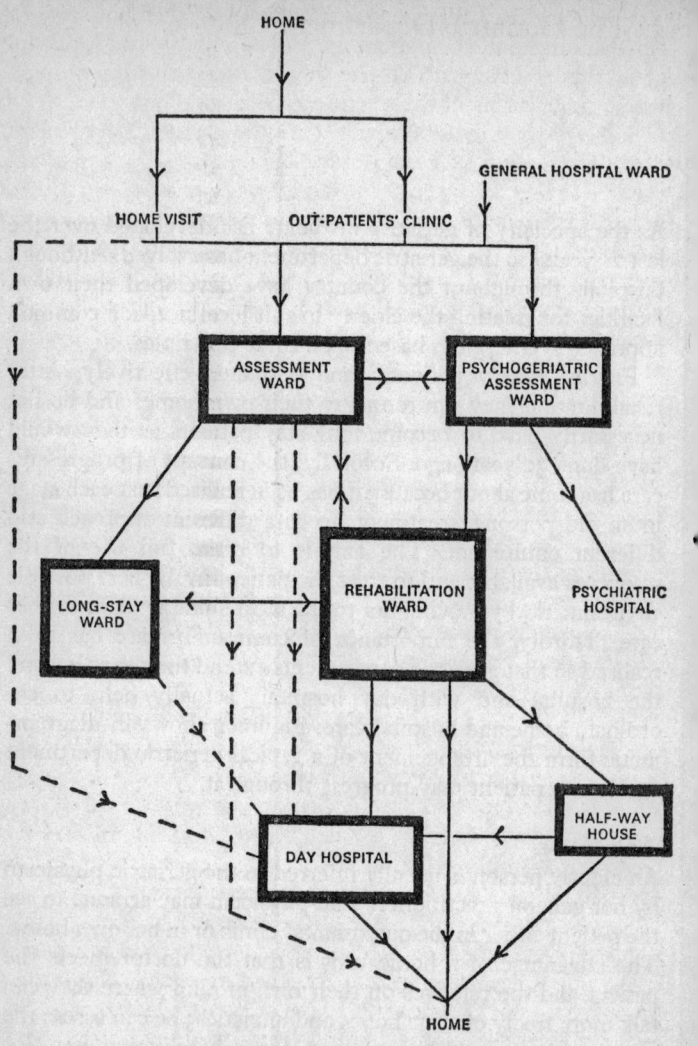

Fig. 1 The Geriatric Department showing the stages of progressive care.

met a doctor from the hospital. As a result of the home visit or clinic assessment, the patient may be admitted as an inpatient or it may be arranged that she should attend the day hospital where some forms of treatment can be carried out.

Some patients will be admitted to the geriatric department direct from other hospital wards. At one time geriatric wards were regarded as dumping grounds for elderly patients from general medical and surgical wards whose prolonged recovery was blocking beds for other admissions. With the growth of geriatric care as a specialty, it is more usual for the patients referred from other wards to be transferred because they have a need for the specialised care, equipment and emphasis on rehabilitation which is not found in general wards. The geriatric physician will assess the patient before transfer in hospital just as he would at home or in the clinic.

The assessment ward

New patients are admitted to the assessment ward for the first few weeks of their stay, where they will be examined, investigations will be undertaken, and any acute illness treated. Their mental state, physical ability and response to rehabilitation will be carefully observed (see Chapter 8), and it may be several weeks before the geriatric team can decide if and when they will be able to return home.

Ideally the assessment ward, the outpatients' department, the day hospital and the rehabilitation ward should all be situated in the district hospital where full diagnostic facilities, such as a comprehensive laboratory service and an X-ray department, are available. To make a full diagnosis it may be necessary for other specialists within the hospital, such as the ophthalmic or orthopaedic surgeons, to be consulted.

Any nurse truly interested in the care of the elderly will, however, undoubtedly sometimes find herself questioning the ethics of submitting certain patients to some diagnostic procedures and treatments. Some investigations can be extremely distressing for an already frail elderly person, and even a fairly straightforward test, which perhaps involves fasting overnight, can be very unpleasant. A patient should not be refused diagnostic facilities available to younger patients on the grounds of age alone yet there must come a time when the value of certain tests and surgical procedures should be weighed against the suffering involved and the probable prognosis, not in terms of survival alone, but in the quality of the life of the patient. While the ultimate decision whether or not a patient should undergo a certain test lies with the doctor, any nurse is justified in voicing her doubts at a ward meeting where the matter can be discussed by all the nursing staff, and the ward sister or charge nurse may wish to express the concern of the nurses to the doctor. This is one way by which an effective ward team, working for the good of the patient in every respect, can be built up, and all the staff can participate in planning the patient's treatment and care.

During their period in the assessment ward, some patients may recover sufficiently to return home, while a few may die. The majority of the remainder will move to the rehabilitation ward. Before any move, the patients and their relatives must be given an explanation for the change of ward and an outline of the treatment to be given there.

The rehabilitation ward

Patients will probably spend most of their time in hospital in the rehabilitation ward. As there will normally be no acutely-ill patients in this ward the staff can direct all their attention to the rehabilitation of the patients (see Chapter 8). In some departments the majority of the patients from the rehabilitation ward will attend the day hospital (see below).

Full use can be made of a dayroom or day area which can be used for meals and activities and so get away from the impression of ill-health implicit in rows of hospital beds. The dayroom is more than a convenient arrangement for gathering all the patients in one place; it is an important part of rehabilitation to keep patients in touch with the life to which they will return so preventing them becoming institutionalised. Old people who are expected to mix socially with other patients will take more trouble over their appearance and will make a greater effort to eat carefully at the communal dining table. During the acute stage of the illness they may be unable to tolerate more than sitting in a chair beside the bed, but once they begin to feel better physically they can become very isolated if their horizons are not extended.

The dayroom should have plenty of visual interest – house plants, a fish tank or a bird in a cage, striking pictures and colourful curtains. The television is often an important focal point as it creates a common interest among the patients and it is a link with the patients' own homes. Chairs should be arranged in groups and not round the walls so that the patients face each other and are not obliged to talk to their neighbours' profile which can make conversation very difficult. Old people are as shy as any other age group and may be nervous of starting a conversation with a complete stranger but the nurse can help by introducing patients to each other with a comment such as 'Mrs C. is a great knitter – she's making a sweater for her grandson', thus introducing two topics of conversation, knitting and the grandson. Deafness makes conversation particularly difficult among the elderly and all patients should be encouraged to wear their hearing aids (see Chapter 6).

Whether or not a dayroom succeeds in being a lively place depends largely on the patients. A nucleus of fairly fit and active patients will stimulate others to be more sociable. Nurses, orderlies and visitors, too, can add to the interest by talking to people either individually or in groups and by letting the patients help with small tasks, like serving tea, looking after the plants and rolling bandages. Men often like to play cards, dominoes or draughts, and jigsaw puzzles attract a small group of enthusiasts. Games, books and magazines, a radio or a record-player should be provided for the patients' use and they should be encouraged to use them. More formal activities may be arranged by the occupational therapist, such as group exercise sessions to music, occupational therapy and painting.

The length of stay in the rehabilitation ward will vary from two weeks to several months, depending on the patients' progress towards independence, which will be helped by the staff's encouragement and enthusiasm.

The day hospital
Geriatric day hospitals are a relatively new concept; the

first was opened in Oxford in the early 1950s, but they were not generally developed until the late 1960s. A day hospital provides all the facilities of the hospital ward except overnight accommodation and is a means of relieving some of the pressure on ward accommodation by providing day care for outpatients who return to their own homes to sleep. A Monday-to-Friday service is usual and patients may attend once, twice or up to five times a week depending on their needs and from about 9.30 a.m. to 4.30 p.m., depending on transport. Psychiatric and psychogeriatric units may also have day hospitals for their outpatients. The geriatric day hospital caters for several categories of patients:

1. The patient who is discharged from the ward to her own home. The rôle of the day hospital in this respect is discussed more fully in Chapter 9.

2. The old person who, although not acutely ill, but for attendance at the day hospital would have had to have been admitted as an inpatient. An example of such a person could be the old lady whose loss of support from friends has led to a deterioration in her physical and mental condition; or the old man whose stroke has left him with hemiplegia and who would benefit from regular exercises in the physiotherapy and occupational therapy departments to improve his mobility.

3. The elderly person who lives at home but would be in hospital if it were not for the care of a relative or friend. Here the day hospital can ease the pressure on those caring for the old person because, by using the facilities of the hospital to treat any medical condition and improve mobility, her total hospitalisation can be prevented or delayed.

The day hospital will have facilities for bathing the patient, washing her clothes, carrying out treatments and dressings; it will provide chiropody and dental care, a hairdressing service, recreational activities and entertainments such as films and outings. There will be a communal dining-room where the provision of a hot mid-day meal may be a crucial factor in allowing a patient to remain at home. Meal times can be an opportunity for the staff to give advice on nutrition, special diets and the preparation of food. The physiotherapy and occupational therapy departments will be situated in or near to the day hospital.

The day hospital has undoubtedly filled a great need and has the added benefit that its convenient hours attract staff more easily. The main problems that arise are usually over the transport of patients to and from their homes. As an ambulance will pick up several patients on each round trip this must inevitably mean a long and tiresome journey for some of the patients, especially those picked up first and set down last, and particularly in crowded urban areas. Where possible a nurse will travel in the ambulance to help the patients and can report if any patient is too ill to attend or if the state of her home appears to be deteriorating.

The halfway house

As its name implies, the halfway house is a small unit where patients can practise living independently under minimal supervision before returning home. Its functions are fully discussed in Chapter 9.

The long-stay ward

About 10 per cent. of all geriatric patients will never be fit enough to return home or even to the sheltered life of an old people's home. These patients will need more nursing care and supervision than old people's homes can give, which can only be provided at present in the long-stay wards of the geriatric department. About one-third to one-half of the beds in a geriatric department will be occupied by long-stay patients and although the condition of a few of these patients may improve sufficiently for them to be discharged, most will remain there for the rest of their lives.

In some geriatric departments the long-stay wards are not in the same hospital as the assessment and rehabilitation wards but may be situated, for example, in an old fever hospital several miles out in the country and inaccessible to elderly relatives. Ideally, there should be a small, long-stay ward in every local hospital in the district. Each ward would still be part of the geriatric department under the supervision of the geriatrician, but the day-to-day medical care may be undertaken by a local general practitioner, preferably the patient's family doctor.

Nursing care in the long-stay ward

The nursing of elderly patients in a long-stay geriatric ward is probably the most demanding work of all and yet it should not be allowed to become a drudgery. Modern aids now available – the Ambu Lift, hoists, ripple beds, water beds, adjustable-height beds and tilting, high-backed chairs (see Chapter 7) – help to make the work less heavy and the nursing care more effective.

Patients who are well enough should be encouraged to get up every day and dress in day clothes in order to spend part of the day in the dayroom or a designated area of the ward. Many of these patients will be incontinent, but efforts to re-train them (Chapter 7) should not be abandoned because they are likely to have to spend the rest of their lives in hospital. Where possible, they should be encouraged to walk to the lavatory or be taken there in a wheelchair at regular times during the day.

Some patients will be mentally confused and noisy but most will want to communicate in some way and will respond to considerate and sensitive care. Each patient should be seen as an individual whose needs are very personal and who must be allowed to live out his or her life with dignity and in comfort. As the emphasis is not on investigations and active treatment the nurse will have more chance to occupy the patient with diversional activities, such as movement games set to music, painting sessions and handicrafts.

How much time is allowed for this sort of activity depends a great deal upon the attitude of individual nurses. It is easy to become so immersed in the arduous routine of getting patients up, feeding them and caring for their physical needs that there seems to be no time for more lighthearted pastimes. Yet these activities are as important a part of the nursing routine as the twice-weekly bath or daily bedmaking. Nurses may go further and actually lighten the burden of caring by making patients interested and alert so that they are more able to help themselves. For instance, each nurse in turn could arrange some entertainment for half an hour every afternoon and watch how each patient responds over a period of a week.

Visitors should be encouraged at all times, but some will

come out of a sense of duty and will be plainly embarrassed after half an hour of awkward conversation. If they, too, can be drawn in to help by entertaining the patients, their visit will become more purposeful and enjoyable. Where the occupational therapist has sufficient help she may be able to spend some time with the long-stay patients and provide them with tasks that make the best use of their handicap and prevent further deterioration. More ambitious projects, such as coach trips, can be arranged, depending on the circumstances of each hospital.

Hospital volunteers, school children, members of the W R V S and other groups, can often help in long-stay wards by befriending a particular patient and perhaps by writing letters, and washing and repairing clothes if the patient has no regular visitors able to do this.

The patients in the long-stay ward

The severely physically disabled. Physically disabled patients who are mentally alert should not be accommodated in the long-stay ward but in a suitable community home, where the constant nursing care they need can be provided, but there is a lamentable shortage of these specialised homes. Such patients will suffer from a variety of crippling diseases – osteoarthritis, rheumatoid arthritis, the after-effects of a stroke, Parkinson's disease, multiple sclerosis and emphysema. Occasionally a very much younger disabled patient will be found in the long-stay ward of a geriatric department because no more suitable place has been found.

These patients make the nursing care in a long-stay ward interesting and rewarding because a close relationship can be built up between nurse and patient. As far as possible the ward should be like home, with the opportunity for the patient to have her own pictures and personal possessions around her. Some severely disabled patients may be able to spend part of the day in the day hospital.

The severely mentally and physically disabled. Many patients who have both mental and physical handicap have suffered a stroke; others may have a crippling disease and a form of dementia. The skill needed to nurse these patients is that of transcending the obvious handicaps and appreciating the patient at her own level of communication. This is particularly so when a patient has little mental disability but great communication difficulty, as in aphasia. It is in the long-stay ward that the nurse has the greatest opportunities to learn to understand some part of the patient's mind and feelings.

Routine care is important so that the patient does not become more confused by too many changes, but routine to the exclusion of any change can make life dull for nurse and patient alike. Moving beds round in the ward can be tried occasionally so that the patient has a different outlook, and changing the position of her chair in the dayroom will help to relieve monotony. However, some severely demented patients are disturbed by any minor alterations to their routine.

The psychogeriatric assessment ward

Some geriatric departments have, in addition to an assessment ward, a psychogeriatric assessment ward to which elderly patients whose main symptoms are some form of disturbed behaviour can be admitted under the care of both the geriatrician and the psychiatrist. Chapter 4 stresses the importance of differentiating between the mental disorders that are amenable to treatment, such as depression and acute toxic confusional states, and the dementias, which are usually progressive disorders.

The joint assessment by both geriatrician and psychiatrist will avoid the dangers of the family doctor having to decide whether a patient is in need of admission to a psychiatric or to a geriatric hospital on the basis of insufficient observation and investigation. The patient suffering from an acute toxic confusional state who is mistakenly admitted to a psychiatric hospital may have the diagnosis of her confusion – heart failure, urinary infection, anaemia – delayed. Once a diagnosis has been made in the psychogeriatric assessment ward, the patient can be treated in the most appropriate place – the patient with dementia in the psychiatric ward or hospital and once treatment has been started the patient with a functional disorder or temporary confusion in the rehabilitation wards of the geriatric department.

The admission of disturbed patients to the psychogeriatric unit will also avoid, to some extent, having noisy patients in the same ward as physically-ill people, who will benefit from a peaceful environment to aid their recovery. The ward can be staffed by nurses who are trained in the care of the mentally ill and who will be better able to understand the patients' needs.

For Further Reading

Brocklehurst, J. C. *Geriatric Day Hospitals*. King Edward's Hospital Fund for London, 1970

Felstein, I. *Later Life: Geriatrics Today and Tomorrow*. Penguin Books, 1969

Norton, D. *Hospitals of the Long-Stay Patient*. Pergamon Press, 1967

Norton, D., Mclaren, R. & Exton-Smith, A. N. *Geriatric Nursing Problems In Hospital*. Churchill-Livingstone, 1975

Robb, B. *Sans Everything, A Case to Answer*. Nelson, 1967

6. Old People as Patients

It has now been established that the patient admitted to a geriatric ward is likely to suffer from several different diseases, to have a degree of physical disability and, possibly, to be mentally confused. Social problems may complicate the picture. Geriatric patients cannot be labelled simply as a case of this or that condition, although, regrettably, this is a habit which lingers in some wards; rather, each patient is an individual who must be treated in a unique fashion, albeit to some general pattern. This approach is as important in the nursing care as it is in the medical treatment.

Two patients' histories which follow illustrate the individual needs of patients who could be mistakenly thought of as being similar cases.

1. 'Mr G., aged 72, a bachelor living alone, is admitted with heart failure, anaemia and acute bronchitis. Until his admission he had felt fit and active and cared for himself. His anaemia and bronchitis are thought to be due to an inadequate diet and to living in a poorly maintained, damp flat. His cardiac failure has occurred as the result of the extra demands made on his heart by the other two conditions. He is anxious to return home to his own, or preferably to another flat in the same area and the aim of treatment is to improve his physical condition as soon as possible and to include in his rehabilitation programme (see Chapter 8) some advice and practical help on cooking and on a more adequate diet. Better accommodation must be sought for him.'

2. 'Mr W., also 72, is a widower who lives with his daughter and her family. He, too, is admitted in cardiac failure and with acute bronchitis. He is a querulous old man whose demands on his daughter have led to unhappiness and conflict within the family and she refuses to have him back. It is unlikely that he will ever manage to live alone and a place in an old people's home seems to be the only solution. He will need to learn to accept this idea and must be encouraged to be

as independent as possible but his very nature may argue against his being able to make the best of the situation. Alternatively, his temperament may improve when away from his family and among his contemporaries and if a place can be found for him he may eventually settle happily into a residential home.'

Elderly people are creatures of habit and when a living pattern of many years is broken on admission to hospital, patients may react by becoming confused, incontinent, aggressive or anorexic. The ward will have its own routine of meal and bed times and once the patients have adapted to their new surroundings their symptoms will often improve. The nurse can help new patients to adapt by constantly reminding them of where they are, why they are there and the date and time of day. Visitors such as doctors or physiotherapists should be clearly introduced and the purpose of the visits explained; new experiences such as a chest X-ray or a blood pressure recording can be very alarming for old people and a simple explanation will prevent unnecessary misunderstanding.

The day to day care of geriatric patients gives the nurse the opportunity to get to know their idiosyncrasies and helps in her understanding of them; this knowledge can be useful when discussing the care of individual patients at ward meetings. It is an effort to talk to old people, especially if they are deaf, but it is unforgivable for staff to discuss personal events such as last night's party with colleagues across the patient while attending to her. If she can be included in the conversation, she will probably respond with some anecdote of her past life which, typically, she will be able to recall vividly. Most people enjoy talking about themselves and any opportunity that will allow the patient to forget the hospital environment for a few minutes is worth pursuing. Elderly people's memories, too, provide a fascinating insight into bygone days. The more the interest shown in a patient, the more will she come to trust the nursing staff and turn to them with her worries. It is a sad fact that the shortage of staff in geriatric wards leaves little time for nurses to sit down and talk to patients, and they are even discouraged from doing this when there is time by the die-hard attitude that expects nurses to be seen to be on the move at all times. Many patients and their relatives seem to imagine that it is wrong to question a doctor or nurse about treatment partly because they always appear to be too busy and so they will ask the most approachable person – the friendly porter or the chatty domestic assistant – and are likely to get an unsatisfactory answer.

Shortage of staff may also mean that the respect for dignity and privacy due to any patient will suffer. Elderly people frequently need help with everything they do and few will openly reproach a nurse for impatient or thoughtless handling – even if they have cause to do so. In wards where there are mentally confused patients it is easy to become lax about privacy, yet it is not for the nurse or anyone else to judge how little a person is aware of her surroundings. Relatives and other patients can also become very distressed by the sight of patients sitting on commodes with curtains undrawn or being walked down the ward with gaping open-backed nightdresses. It is the duty of every nurse to safeguard the dignity of her patients, however confused they may be, and to treat them with the thoughtfulness due to anyone in the care of others and as they themselves would wish to be treated in similar circumstances. Patients will respond to this attention by becoming more sociable in their habits and brighter in mood.

Encouraging independence is another important aspect of the general care of the elderly, for many patients will return home, some to homes that are unsuitable and others to live alone (see Chapter 9). The nurse is in a strong position to encourage independence, to applaud every effort that the patient makes and to accept that the price of independence may be spilt food, aggravatingly slow movements, especially when dressing, and even occasional falls. Rather than restraining patients, it is better to prevent accidents by showing them the best way to get out of bed and how to use the walking frame correctly, and to provide them with suitable aids and utensils (see Chapter 8).

Confused or demented patients
Many patients in the geriatric ward will suffer some form of

mental disorder (see Chapter 4), and one of the nurse's more difficult tasks is to learn to treat them with the same consideration and respect she would treat a well-orientated, alert patient. One of the reasons for tactless and thoughtless handling of a mentally disturbed patient is the nurse's embarrassment at not knowing how best to approach her.

Firstly, it is important to try to understand the patient's behaviour. Unfortunately, mental disorders cannot be diagnosed as quickly and accurately as, for instance, iron-deficiency anaemia, but if the nurse is aware of the possible causes of the patient's behaviour, her own observations may help in the diagnosis.

Secondly, the patients should be treated as far as possible in the same way as mentally alert people. They may not understand the explanation of a procedure but will appreciate the reassurance in the tone of voice used and simple physical contact of holding their hand. There is no reason why mentally disordered patients should not be allowed the same privacy as alert patients; they will be at no less risk of falling because their cubicle curtains have been left open while they are getting dressed or sitting on a commode. If their changes in behaviour are anticipated and movements are carefully supervised accidents can be prevented. If a patient is using a commode by the bed and the nurse has to leave to attend to other patients, the commode should be turned to face the bed, which must have its wheels braked, so that if the patient tries to stand and support herself, she will at least fall onto the bed. Preferably, a nurse should remain with the patient if there is a danger that she may fall.

Aimiably demented patients. Old persons who are aimiably demented can usually be tolerated in the general ward without causing too much disruption. They will probably be suffering from a form of dementia which may have been apparent for some time before admission to hospital for another condition, such as an acute chest infection. Relatives may describe them as being muddled and forgetful at home and their confusion may increase when confronted with the strange environment and unusual routine of the hospital. After an initial few days of agitation and confusion, aimiably demented patients should settle down and be able to do much for themselves. They may appear to live in a world of their own but provided they do not endanger themselves or others there is no reason why they should not be allowed to do as they wish, even if it means packing and repacking their suitcases several times a day. Efforts to restrain them or to try to make them conform to an accepted pattern of behaviour will merely increase their agitation.

Drugs such as cyclandelate (Cyclospasmal) which increase the blood supply to the brain may be ordered by the doctor to help make a patient less confused. Tranquillisers, such as chlorpromazine (Largactil), promazine (Sparine) and perphenazine (Fentazine) may improve the agitation and decrease the restlessness but increase the confusion. If the patient is allowed to be sufficiently active during the day and is not expected to go to bed too early, night sedation may be unnecessary (see Sleep, p. 89).

Delirious patients. One of the more difficult tasks in the nursing of old people is the care and control of delirious patients. Acute toxic confusional states or senile dementia (see Chapter 4) can each be the cause of a patient becoming severely confused, disorientated, agitated, violent and noisy. The problems are how to restrain patients to prevent them hurting themselves, but not so severely as to increase their distress, and how to limit the amount of disruption such patients will cause in the ward.

If the patient is anoxic, oxygen given by Ventimask for short periods will help to increase the oxygen supply to the brain and so lessen the confusion, although the mask may increase the patient's agitation. Dehydration can be a factor contributing to the acute confusional state and the patient may be persuaded to take glucose drinks or sweetened tea. Intravenous infusions or fluids by naso-gastric tube are unlikely to be tolerated by the delirious patient. Pain, discomfort from a pressure sore, a full bladder or constipation can increase the patient's agitation. The nursing staff who constantly observe the patient are in a position to recognise and alleviate possible causes of distress and the ward team can discuss the best method of management. Sedative drugs are not given as a matter of course to elderly delirious patients because in a state of sedation they are likely to become anoxic and at greater risk of developing broncho-pneumonia through immobility. Sedation may also mask the signs and symptoms of acute physical illness. The medications most likely to be used in extreme cases are chloral hydrate, paraldehyde or chlorpromazine. Barbiturates are not given to elderly people as they increase their confusion.

When possible, delirious patients should be nursed in a single room or in a part of the ward where the noise will least disturb other patients. They should be surrounded by their familiar possessions – dressing gown, handbag – and the light should be left on at night. The nurse should approach the patient calmly, using her name and explaining what she is going to do. Shouting at the patient who does not seem to understand will only increase the patient's confusion.

Restraining the delirious patient poses problems which should not be underestimated. Apparently frail old ladies become incredibly strong when delirious, perhaps needing two or three nurses to hold them, and, especially at night, there may not be this number of staff available. However, to restrain patients by tying down their arms or by using cot sides is not the easy solution in a staff shortage; such methods are likely to increase agitation as they try to resist the restraints and in doing so may injure themselves and create more disturbance. If they are allowed within reason to do as they wish – to get out of bed, sit in a chair, walk round the ward – they will become less violent. It will be necessary for at least one nurse to be with such a patient continually at this time to reassure, not by denying or ridiculing any delusions but by accepting them and then diverting the patient's attention from them.

Relatives are often particularly distressed by the sight of an old person behaving aggressively, especially when it appears to be a personal attack on them. If they have had to cope with the old person in this state before admission to hospital, they will be relieved to relinquish their responsibility, but a very close relative may be prepared to spend some time with the patient during the acute confusional state, so long as she has the support and guidance of the nursing staff who can take a more detached view of the patient's condition.

Depressed patients. Depression (see Chapter 4) is difficult to diagnose in the elderly, and in a busy ward apathetic patients who make no effort to help themselves, or the agitated patients who baulk every attempt to be helped, may not get the attention they need. It is obviously essential that depressed patients should be diagnosed accurately but it is easy for a patient's behaviour to be accepted by all the staff and it may need a newcomer to the ward to ask why a certain patient does not do more for herself when it appears she could. Relatives may also be able to point to a change in behaviour or remember a previous occasion when the patient has been psychologically disturbed.

Once depression has been diagnosed and treatment started, the nursing staff are in the best position to assess the effectiveness of the treatment. Anti-depressant drugs take several days to take effect and the change in the patient's behaviour will be gradual. On becoming more responsive the patient should be given every encouragement to do a little more, such as washing the face and hands and feeding – the basic tasks of personal care. Her social background will need careful investigation by the social worker so that any particular problems that may have contributed to the depression, can be remedied.

Mental testing

Many geriatric departments make use of a simple oral test to assess each patient on admission and to gauge various aspects of mental ability including short- and long-term memory, orientation in time and space and powers of concentration. The patient is asked simple questions by the doctor or nurse conducting the test; for example, the time of day, the place, the date of the Second World War and the name of the Prime Minister, to recite numbers forward and backwards, and is also given a short address to remember and recall after a few minutes. The person conducting the test should give the patient a simple explanation of its purpose; for instance: 'Mrs C., the doctor likes to test the memory of all our new patients. Perhaps you have found your memory has not been so good lately. I would like to ask you some questions but do not worry if you cannot answer them.' Some alert patients may feel insulted by being asked simple questions, but many elderly people hesitate and find difficulty with apparently quite simple tasks like counting backwards. The questions must be asked in a clear voice and if the patient is deaf, a card with the questions printed on it may be used. The resulting score of the test given on admission can then be compared with one repeated after ten days, or any other suitable period.

The results of these tests can be very interesting. In the case of patients admitted suffering from an acute toxic confusional state, the score of the first test is likely to be very low, but as their physical condition improves so will their mental state and the test score after a week or ten days will be much higher. Patients whose test score is low on admission and do no better, or even worse after ten days despite an improvement in their physical condition, may be suffering from a form of dementia. Depressed patients should be able to answer the questions reasonably easily despite being withdrawn and agitated; however, they may refuse to answer and their score after treatment has started will be a guide to its effectiveness in improving their condition.

Sleep and confusion in patients at night
Many elderly people are poor sleepers and may only sleep for short periods. At home they will have their own methods of coping with insomnia; by going to bed late, getting up early, reading for periods or even walking round the house in the middle of the night and making themselves a cup of tea. Unfortunately, the hospital situation rarely allows for these habits. Patients are usually expected to be in bed by the time the day staff leave the ward at eight or nine o'clock, and although they are often woken early, they will not be permitted to wander round during the night or turn on a light to read a book.

Night nurses often report that a patient who is normally well-orientated during the day has become very confused at night. This may be because they have become muddled by waking up in a strange place, and a dimmed light should be left on to help them to become familiar with their surroundings. A cup of tea is often appreciated during a wakeful period and patients may find re-assurance in a nurse sitting by their bed. However, a more likely cause for confusion at night is unnecessary sedation. A sedative may be offered as a matter of course to all elderly patients to help them to cope with the long night, and most will accept it. Those unused to sleeping pills will sleep more deeply than normal and will wake befuddled. Nocturnal frequency is particularly common in elderly people and if patients try to get up hurriedly in a drowsy state, they may fall. They may find, too, that they have been incontinent, because they have been too deeply asleep to respond to the urge to pass urine. Drug-induced sleep will, unfortunately, often cause more problems than it solves.

To cope with the problems of night-time confusion, night nurses must accept that elderly people are often restless and wakeful and that, therefore, they are likely to require as much nursing care as they would during the day. If patients are encouraged to be as active as possible during the day and their bed times are flexible, there should be no need to give night sedation to those who are not accustomed to it.

However, wakeful patients may be made more comfortable if they are allowed to sit out of bed for a short time to ease their stiffened joints – an exercise as valuable as the routine 'two-hourly turn'. Some patients are shy of asking for help to move or to use a bedpan and may lie uncomfortably because they do not want to disturb the nurse!

The use of cot sides. One of the least attractive sights in a geriatric hospital is to see a row of beds with all the patients hedged in by cot sides. It is a practical expression of the attitude that equates old age with second childhood and damages the dignity of the old person. Cot sides have a place in geriatric wards, as in any other ward, but they should not be looked upon as a universal solution by overworked nursing staff, particularly at night. The indiscriminate use of cot sides can be dangerous because a patient who climbs over a cot side and falls is likely to suffer more harm than one who falls out of a normal bed where the fall may be broken by the restraining bedclothes.

The main use of cot sides is to stop a patient from FALLING out of bed: they should not be used to stop a patient from

GETTING out of bed. They are necessary for restless patients who are unconscious or semi-conscious, and those who have had a stroke may feel more secure at night if the cot side is up along the edge of the bed to which they have a tendency to gravitate. Frail patients may also find reassurance in the security of cot sides.

Nurses may feel tempted to put cot sides on the beds of patients known to be confused or to wander at night to prevent them from getting out, but if such patients should wake with an urge to pass urine their first instinct will be to try to get out of bed and in doing so, may climb over the cot side and fall. If they realise that they are hemmed in and cannot get out they may resign themselves to becoming incontinent. The night staff need to be especially vigilant so that they are instantly aware of patients who are restless and can go to their aid with a bedpan or commode before an accident occurs.

It is doubtful if cot sides are helpful in restraining extremely delirious patients, for they, too, may try to climb over them; cot sides also prevent the nurse from reaching patients easily. The best kind of cot sides are those that are fixed to the bed rail and will fold away under the bed so that the nursing staff do not have to struggle to fit and remove them. The nurse should never attempt to lift or turn a patient while the cot sides are up as she will risk straining her back.

Deaf patients

Deaf or partially deaf patients are common in geriatric wards because so many elderly people suffer some hearing loss, but people working with the elderly must guard against raising their voices to every elderly person, as it is easy to fall into the habit of assuming, incorrectly, that all old people are deaf.

Deafness can hinder successful rehabilitation because the patient cannot grasp quickly the instructions and advice given. It also makes casual conversation between patients very difficult and probably accounts for the lack of interaction between them.

How to talk to the elderly deaf

Deaf people not only lose their hearing but sounds become

distorted and loud sounds, particularly, are aggravating. A deaf person should be spoken to slowly in a slightly raised voice with the words clearly enunciated. Some people can lip read and may understand more than is realised so it is important for the speaker to be in a good light and facing the patient so that her mouth can be seen. If the patient does not at first understand, the sentence may be reworded to make it clearer. Conversation can be elaborated by the use of simple actions and facial expressions – a shake of the head, a clap of the hands for approval. Other noises may distract the old person and should be eliminated as far as possible to encourage concentration on the speaker.

It may be simpler for a very deaf person and less frustrating for the speaker if the conversation is written and such a patient can be provided with a pad and pencil for the purpose.

Hearing aids. The hearing aids provided by the National Health Service and worn on the body, will help the patient to hear direct conversation but cannot restore the full sense of hearing. This limitation must be explained to the patient, who otherwise may quickly discard the aid because she feels she can hear no better with it. Various points are important in the use of these aids.

1. The earpiece is moulded to fit the wearer's ear and it will not fit another person. A whistling noise may be due to a poorly fitting ear piece which allows sound to escape from the ear.

2. The batteries will need to be changed regularly and must be fitted in the correct way. A supply of new batteries should be kept on the ward.

3. The easiest way to talk to a patient wearing an aid is to sit facing her and holding the microphone (the box part of the aid) in the hand, speaking into it in a normal, clear voice. When the person moves about the aid should be clipped to the clothing with the microphone facing forward and not covered.

Hearing aids which fit behind the ear will eventually replace the National Health Service box type aid, but at present such aids can only be bought privately. It is important that they should be fitted by a qualified practitioner as one type of aid may be less suitable than another. These aids are generally more acceptable because they are less bulky and obtrusive and depend less upon the microphone being pointed in a particular direction.

Speaking tubes and trumpets are mechanical means of amplifying sound without distortion. The speaking tube has a two-inch wide mouthpiece and a flexible tube three feet long with an ear piece at the other end; it can be very effective for direct conversation. The ear trumpet is still found by some people to be the best way of listening to someone talking directly to them as it concentrates the sound to one point. A similar effect is gained by cupping the hand round the ear and turning towards the speaker.

There is a danger that deaf people can become isolated, perhaps less so in their own homes, where at least the people around them will be aware of their deafness, than in hospital where demands upon staff are heavy and there is little time to talk to the deaf patient other than on essential matters. Talking to deaf people involves extra effort and patience. Deaf people do not have the auditory clues that people of normal hearing take for granted; they wake in the morning and cannot tell the time from the clatter of the early morning tea trolley and they may only be aware of the doctor's round when he stands in front of them. More than most patients they will need nurses and other staff to remind them of the time of day, where they are and why they are there so that they do not get disorientated. Even when patients have a hearing aid it takes a little effort on everyone's part to encourage them to use it and not let it be tucked away in the locker drawer so that they have to be content with a minimum of conversation.

Blind patients

Many elderly people have poor sight, which in some cases can be improved by the use of spectacles and in others by a cataract operation or other treatment. People who go blind later in life can often manage to live satisfactorily in their own homes where the surroundings are familiar but may have not developed the skill of using a stick and finding their way around a new place. Elderly blind patients will need considerable help and guidance in the ward, particularly when they have other disabilities such as deafness or restricted movement.

Some patients may never venture from their chairs without a guiding hand, while others having learned the geography of the ward may manage to walk to the lavatory using the handrails.

It is most important to remember that blind people have no means of knowing who is approaching them until something is said. It is unforgivable to go up to a blind person with, for instance, a meal tray, put it down in front of her without a word and walk away. Anything that is to be done for the patient must be explained beforehand, but not just 'Mrs B., we are going to give you a bath' as she is wheeled briskly down the ward; far better, 'Mrs B., this is Nurse N. Nurse C. and I would like to give you a bath in about ten minutes when we have finished helping Mrs D'.

Blind persons should be expected to help themselves with some of the activities of daily living (see Chapter 8) such as washing and dressing and feeding. The blind, unlike the deaf, arouse considerable compassion and it is a great temptation to help when patients are seen to be fumbling to do up their buttons, but if the aim is for the patients to become as independent as possible they must be given suitable aids and allowed to manage by themselves, once they are fit enough. An old person may be unable to learn the technique of using a stick, but a walking frame will not only be a support but will also act as a solid guide to obstacles in an unfamiliar place.

Some blind and partially-sighted people who are not registered with their local authority may not realise the benefits of being so registered. To be registered as blind or partially sighted the person has to be referred by her doctor for a special examination by an ophthalmologist. A person who is registered is entitled to a special tax allowance, to a higher rate of supplementary pension and to a television licence at a reduced rate. There are also certain travel concessions.

A registered blind person will be visited by a social worker, and will be able to attend local clubs and specially arranged activities, as well as meeting other blind people through the local welfare committee for the blind, which will be affiliated to the Royal National Institute for the Blind. The person will also be able to hire a 'talking book' and borrow tapes for it, and may be lent a radio or radio headphones.

Care of the dying

The emphasis of this book is directed towards the rehabilitative aspect of geriatric care but it would be unrealistic not to stress the importance of the care of the dying patient. As in any ward there will come a time in the care of some patients when active treatment must give way to palliative care, particularly in the long-stay wards. It may be this aspect of geriatric care which makes it unattractive to many nurses but death in the geriatric ward must be seen in perspective.

Firstly, the death of an old person has less of the tragedy of the death of a child or young adult, when the circumstances of their dying is likely to be traumatic with extremely grieved relatives attending the patient or with heroic attempts at resuscitation. Rarely is it necessary to attempt to resuscitate elderly people and the onus is on the doctors and nurses to allow patients to die with dignity and in peace. Secondly, many elderly people are ready to die. They have seen their contemporaries die, their recent life may have been difficult and lonely. Sometimes they feel out of step with the speed and fashions of the modern world. Many will say, 'I am ready to die, why should I go on living.'

The problem in the geriatric ward is, perhaps, not to allow the death of a patient to be taken as a matter of course. The attitude of the nurses will be closely observed by the other patients and their relatives, who will naturally be distressed by any apparently casual treatment of death. The junior nurse may not always receive from senior staff the guidance she should expect on the most appropriate manner to cope with death, nor is it a subject that can easily be learnt from a book or in the classroom. Her behaviour should be naturally composed without being unnecessarily distant, and compassionate without being sentimental.

Death is the one event in life that cannot be made easier to understand by drawing on the experience of others, and the approach to it is a highly individual experience related to the patient's way of life. Elderly people have had time to consider and in some way come to terms with their own death, either by accepting its inevitability or by filling their minds with other thoughts in order to avoid dwelling on it. Most people find difficulty in expressing their deepest feelings and fears, and some may be able to talk more easily to a comparative stranger than to a relative or friend. Sadly, traditional attitudes and a lack of guidance in the art of counselling means that few nurses are able to sit down and talk to their patients, and lack of privacy and patients' deafness may, in any case, make intimate conversation difficult.

Some patients will find strength and comfort in their religion, even if they have not been practising members of a church for years, and the hospital chaplain or their own minister can be of great support at this time. Fear is probably the predominant emotion of dying people – fear of the unknown, fear of being left alone, fear of being the cause of unhappiness and fear of behaving inappropriately. The nurse must use all her powers of observation and compassion to sense how the patient is coping with these fears.

If the nurse should be confronted by a patient who asks about her approaching death she should try to answer as honestly as possible without resorting to clichés and platitudes. If she feels she cannot cope with such questions and the patient is distressed, she should ask the senior nurses for advice and help. It is helpful if the nurses, doctors and paramedical staff have agreed on a common approach to the patient who is dying so that misunderstandings do not arise and the patient and her relatives are not given conflicting information.

The nurse is likely to encounter more dying patients during her time in the geriatric ward than in any other part of her experience, and for the conscientious nurse this could be an overwhelming burden but for the fact that many elderly people die suddenly or death is preceded by a period of unconsciousness. It is unlikely that these patients have been acutely troubled by thoughts of approaching death and the nurse's responsibility is for their physical comfort without the stress of having to give spiritual relief.

Practical care
The practical care should be directed towards making the

dying patient as comfortable as possible, and free from distressing symptoms. The doctor should be asked to discontinue any treatment or drugs that can no longer be of any help to the patient; a dying person should not be expected to swallow iron tablets or a routine aperient merely because at one time they were prescribed for her. When the patient shows signs of discomfort, the answer is not necessarily heavy sedation, which will increase the risk of pressure sores and further discomfort; the causes of the discomfort should be sought and as far as possible, alleviated. Among the main causes of discomfort are the following:

(a) Restlessness. There are many reasons why a patient may be restless, the more important of which are:

Pain, a frequent cause of restlessness, is considered in detail below.

Anoxia. Lack of oxygen to the brain will make the patient confused and restless. Oxygen given by mask may increase the supply to the brain but the mask itself may make the patient more distressed. Oxygen can be given intermittently following the administration of a sedative such as chlorpromazine.

Thirst. Thirst can make a patient feel very uncomfortable. A dry mouth will quickly become sore and regular mouth toilet will be appreciated. Sips of water or fruit juice, sufficient to moisten the mouth, may be all that the patient can manage. Where dehydration is severe an intravenous infusion or fluids given by naso-gastric tube may be tried to relieve the restlessness.

Patients should be permitted to eat and drink whatever they wish and need not have high protein food and drinks pressed upon them on the pretext that they are good for them; the adage 'a little of what you fancy does you good' seems appropriate here. Patients who cannot manage any solid food may appreciate an egg flip (raw egg beaten in milk with a little sugar and, perhaps, a little brandy) and a plain biscuit to nibble.

Bladder care. A distended bladder will cause discomfort and restlessness but may not immediately be recognised if the patient has retention of urine with overflow and constantly dribbles small quantities; the distended bladder will be felt as a mass above the symphysis pubis. Catheterization will be necessary to relieve the pressure and discomfort.

Bowel care. Constipation can cause discomfort and restlessness. Inactive patients taking only small quantities of fluid may have a very hard stool which they cannot pass. The least traumatic way to relieve this condition is to give the patient an olive oil enema to be retained for twelve hours, followed by a small evacuant enema.

Renal failure. A degree of renal failure is common in the dying and in severe cases can cause distressing restlessness, hiccoughing and vomiting. Sedatives such as chlorpromazine and pethidine may be ordered to help to relieve these symptoms.

(b) Pain. The dying patient can suffer pain from terminal disease, such as a carcinoma, or from a secondary condition, such as arthritis or a pressure sore. Pain in the elderly is not usually such a dominating symptom in terminal disease as it is in a younger patient. Nevertheless, if a patient complains of pain, effective drugs should not be withheld for fear the patient may become dependent on them. Analgesic drugs for terminal pain should be carefully calculated and given at regular intervals BEFORE the pain occurs so that the patient is spared the anticipation of pain. In this way the dose of the drug can be kept to the minimum; even mild analgesics such as paracetamol and codeine, if given regularly, may be sufficient. A mild sedative drug, such as small doses of chlorpromazine can be used to reduce the patient's tension and ease anxiety. The nurse is in the best position to judge the effectiveness of the analgesia prescribed and it is her responsibility to see that it is given regularly. Pain from arthritic joints and pressure sores can be relieved if the patient's position is altered regularly and she may feel easier if she can sit out of bed in a chair for a short period.

(c) Breathlessness. Severe dyspnoea, resulting from pulmonary congestion which occurs in cardiac and respiratory failure, is a common symptom of distress in the dying. Not only is it extremely distressing for the patient to be fighting ineffectively for every breath, but it is very upsetting for the relatives to watch.

Positioning is obviously important; therefore, to ease distress the patient should either be propped up, well supported by a back rest and pillows, or be nursed in a cardiac bed, or she may even find it more comfortable to sit in a chair. Sitting upright will relieve abdominal pressure on the lungs and allow for their greatest expansion. Oxygen in low concentration may help in some cases but the mask can increase a sense of suffocation. Morphia or pethidine given by intramuscular injection is effective and if ordered should be administered regularly.

(d) Nausea and vomiting occur in the terminal stages of many conditions and can be extremely distressing symptoms. An anti-emetic drug such as promazine (Sparine) will usually help. Regular mouth toilet will help the patient to feel fresher and relieve thirst.

A daily bed-bath, regular sponging of the face and hands and frequent turning can be soothing, even for the semi-conscious patient, and will help to control restlessness. These and similar nursing procedures are often more effective than sedatives in terminal care and underline how much the truly effective care of the dying is dependent upon nursing skills. Many of the symptoms of distress in the dying are compounded by anxiety and fear and the nurse can relieve much of this fear by her presence and her sympathetic handling of the patient as well as the intuitive anticipation of her needs.

The patient's relatives

An important part of the task of nursing the dying is the support of the patient's relatives. Whenever possible, close relatives should be allowed to stay with a dying person at all reasonable times because their presence will be a great comfort. Relatives may have ambivalent feelings about the patient's death: on the one hand they will feel relieved that there is soon to be an end to suffering and they will be released from the responsibility of care, and on the other they will feel deeply grieved at losing someone they love. They may fear that their lack of demonstrative grief is a sign of callousness and worry that their sense of relief may be misconstrued. Such reactions are normal and relatives can be reassured if they express their uncertainty. A more overwhelming sense of grief often comes later when they physically miss the dead person.

It happens occasionally that an old person has been the cause of some family controversy and the death-bed becomes the scene of bitter family rows over money or property. When this happens in hospital, great care must be taken by the ward sister and doctors that the patient's relatives are allowed reasonable access but that the patient is not unnecessarily upset and that the arguments do not take place in the ward. It is difficult for an outsider to judge the true reasons behind family dissension and it is safer not to become involved.

Practical aspects of death
Wills. A nurse may be asked to witness a patient's signature to a will. Anyone who is not a beneficiary of the will can legally witness the signature but if, as occasionally happens, a dispute over the will arises, it may be said that the nurse had undue influence over the patient. A nurse who is asked to witness a will should refer the request to the ward sister for the attention of the hospital administration department who will follow the legal procedure laid down by the National Health Service.

Death certificate. The certificate will be given to the next-of-kin of the deceased person. It will be signed by the doctor who treated the patient in hospital and will state the cause of death and any other condition that may have contributed to it. Unless a post-mortem examination is to be carried out (see below) it is usual for a relative to be asked to return to the hospital on the day after the death to collect the certificate and the deceased person's possessions. The death certificate must then be taken to the offices of the Registrar of Births, Deaths and Marriages for the district in which the hospital is situated.

Registration. A death must be registered within five days and the Registrar will give the relative a certificate (known as the disposal certificate) which authorises the undertaker to arrange for the burial of the body. If the body is to be cremated a further certificate is required from the Registrar and this is signed by an independent doctor and the doctor attending the crematorium.

The death grant. Most people will, by virtue of their own or their husband's National Insurance Contributions, be eligible for the Death Grant (£30 in 1975) which is paid to the deceased person's next-of-kin within three months of the death and is intended to help towards funeral expenses. A form for applying for this grant is given to the person registering the death.

Post mortem examination. A post mortem examination to determine the cause of death and other contributory conditions is legally necessary in certain cases and is considered advisable if there is any doubt. If a patient dies within 24 hours of admission, dies suddenly and unexpectedly, dies during or soon after an operation, or dies following an accident, such as a fall, a post-mortem examination will be performed. The coroner of the district will be told if a post-mortem examination has been carried out and he will order an inquest if he is not satisfied that the death was from natural causes. When a post-mortem examination has been performed for any of the foregoing reasons, the coroner will issue the death certificate. In most cases he will authorise the funeral to take place before the inquest is held and the final certificate issued.

Occasionally, the doctor will ask the deceased patient's relatives for permission to carry out a post-mortem examination when there is no legal necessity but when it would be of medical interest, and the relatives can refuse if they wish. However, it should be explained to them that research is important and much can be learned about disease and the process of ageing from regular post-mortem examinations of geriatric patients. The coroner is not involved and the funeral can take place without delay.

For Further Reading

Bromley, D. B. *The Psychology of Human Ageing*. Penguin Books, 1966

Rudinger, E. *What to Do when Someone Dies*. Consumers Association, 1972

Saunders, C. *Care of the Dying*. *Nursing Times* Reprint, 1960

How to talk to the Elderly Deaf. London Borough of Haringey, 1970

7. Aspects of Nursing Care

Caring for the elderly patient gives the nurse an opportunity to develop further certain aspects of those fundamental skills taught her at the beginning of training and practised by her in the general wards.

1. Pressure sores

The prevention of pressure sores is considered to be one criterion of good geriatric nursing and it reflects badly on the standard of nursing care if a patient develops a sore while in the ward. The 'back-round' has become an inescapable part of the ward routine, yet in many cases the regular wash and rub with cream is unnecessary and if badly done, is ineffective or may even be harmful. Pressure sores are seen in geriatric wards, usually because patients are admitted with them but even in the busiest of wards, sores should not develop if all resources are concentrated on preventing their occurrence in patients most at risk.

(a) The cause of pressure sores

It is important to understand why pressure sores develop. They can occur in any part of the body where a bone lies closely under the skin and which is subjected to prolonged though not necessarily heavy pressure, or where the skin and subcutaneous tissue are dragged or sheared over the underlying muscle and bone by the weight of the body. A healthy person does not suffer from pressure sores because prolonged pressure causes discomfort which makes him change position frequently, even when he is asleep. His skin is normally resistant to pressure and shearing forces because it is strong, elastic and protected from moisture by its own oils. Pressure sores are more likely to occur where the skin has become friable through being soaked with urine or where oedema has formed, such as around the sacral area of patients with cardiac failure who are confined to bed. Patients who are anaemic or poorly nourished are at greater risk of developing sores and broken devitalised skin will take longer to heal. Particularly vulnerable areas occur over the sacrum, the greater trocanters, the ischial tuberosities, the heels, the inner aspect of the knees and shins, the elbows and the scapulae.

There are two types of pressure sore.

Superficial sores. A superficial sore starts as a small abrasion of the skin in a vulnerable area. Pressure on the area causes thromboses to form in the small blood vessels supplying the skin and subcutaneous tissues, oedema forms, the blood supply is severely restricted, the abrasion cannot heal and the surrounding skin and tissue breaks down creating a larger, superficial sore which can be very painful. If this type of sore is treated effectively at an early stage and the pressure is relieved (see below) the blood supply will improve and the area will heal.

Deep sores. Deep pressure sores develop insidiously beneath the skin, and are caused by pressure and by shearing of the skin and subcutaneous tissue away from the deeper structures, causing damage to the blood vessels supplying the area, which quickly becomes necrosed. The skin will at first remain intact although it may look dark red and bruised, but when finally it breaks down the necrotic area beneath may be very extensive and deep, and even expose the bone. If the area becomes infected the necrosis may spread further and healing will be delayed.

The patients most likely to develop sores are those who
1. are unable to move themselves to relieve pressure, e g the hemiplegic, the very obese and those with respiratory or severe cardiac failure;
2. cannot feel the discomfort of prolonged pressures, e g the unconscious and semi-conscious, the confused and the paraplegic;
3. are incontinent of urine and faeces; and
4. are anaemic, poorly nourished, very ill or frail.

The burden of care in the geriatric ward can be relieved by identifying those patients most liable to develop sores and concentrating measures to relieve pressure and to protect the vulnerable areas of these patients. A table has been devised* to assess the liability of patients to develop pressure sores by scoring points against five aspects of their condition, thus:

A Physical cond.		B Mental state		C Activity		D Mobility		E Incontinence	
Good	4	Alert	4	Ambulant	4	Full	4	None	4
Fair	3	Apathetic	3	Walk/help	3	Sl. limited	3	Occasional	3
Poor	2	Confused	2	Chair-bound	2	Very limited	2	Usually of urine	2
Very bad	1	Stuporose	1	Bedfast	1	Immobile	1	Double	1

Those patients scoring more than 14 are *unlikely* to develop pressure sores *unless* their condition deteriorates, but with a score of 14 or below, they are liable to develop sores; a score below 12 makes the *risk very great* indeed. All patients should be reassessed on alternate days and the score recorded in their daily report or other suitable place. Use of the scoring system does not mean that patients scoring more than 14 are neglected. At night they will need to be made comfortable, to have their pillows and sheets straightened and their pressure areas examined for signs of redness, but time during the day which would have been spent in preventive treatment can be better used to help such patients to regain their independence.

The following example shows how two patients might be assessed.

'Mrs A., aged 76, who is very obese, has been admitted in cardiac failure. She is an apathetic old lady who has suffered from severe osteo-arthritis for several years. She has occasionally been incontinent of urine but is frequently so when given diuretics. She would score as follows: physical condition 2; mental state 3; activity 2; mobility 2; incontinence 2 = total 11. Mrs A. is therefore at very great risk of developing pressure sores and preventive measures must be taken. She should

---

* Norton D., Mclaren R. & Exton-Smith A.N. (1962, reprinted 1976). *An Investigation of Geriatric Nursing Problems in Hospital*

be helped regularly to alter her position and *must* be kept clean and dry, her sheets being changed as soon as they are wet. As her incontinence and mobility improve she will still be liable to develop sores, but the risk will be less great.'

'Mr L., aged 82, is also in cardiac failure following an attack of acute bronchitis exacerbating his chronic bronchitic condition. He is a slightly-built active man, despite a stroke four years previously which left him with slight residual hemiplegia. He would score: physical condition 3; mental state 4; activity 3; mobility 3; incontinence 4 total 17. Mr L. is alert and active and is therefore unlikely to develop pressure sores, but the elbow and heel on his affected side should be examined for signs of pressure and massaged every day.'

(b) *The treatment of pressure areas to prevent sores*

Having identified the patients who are at risk it is necessary to understand the principles which govern the prevention of pressure sores.

(i) **Relief of pressure by altering the patient's position.**

All patients who are unconscious, semi-conscious, very ill, confused or unable to move themselves should have their position changed two-hourly, by day and night. It takes skill and ingenuity to turn a patient with the minimum of disturbance and it is easier with three rather than two nurses (see Turning the Patient, page 127). The patient should never be dragged up the bed, because this will cause shearing of the skin over the bony sacrum and seriously damage the underlying tissues, but must be lifted clear of the bed by two nurses using the Australian lift (see p. 126) while the third nurse pulls the draw sheet through, straightens the undersheet and sweeps it free of debris.

It is tempting to think that those patients who are not nursed in bed are free from the risk of pressure sores, at least while they are up, but relatively immobile patients who spend their day sitting in a chair are likely to develop sores over their ischial tuberosities if the pressure is not relieved regularly. If such patients are helped to stand and walk a few steps every hour, or if their chair is moved to the end of the bed where they can pull themselves up by the bed-rail (see p. 137 for end of bed exercises), not only will pressure be relieved but the blood supply to the area will be improved by exercise.

(ii) **Aids for the relief of pressure.** There are various mechanical aids for relieving pressure but these cannot replace entirely the need to alter the patient's position regularly. The *Ripple bed*, or alternating pressure mattress, has an electric motor which pumps air into alternate sections of the mattress during a five to ten-minute cycle. The large cell variety is the most useful because it can be maintained at a sufficiently high pressure to keep the patient clear of the bed. The pressure is altered according to the patient's weight and care must be taken to see that the air inlets have not become detached from the motor and that the motor is running. Ripple beds add several inches to the height of the normal hospital bed and make nursing more difficult so that where possible the bed should be lowered to a convenient height.

The *water mattress* is a recent development based on a well-tried principle. The patient lies on a mattress filled with water so that the pressure is evenly spread beneath the body. While these mattresses help to solve the pressure problem, the patient, particularly an older one, may find it difficult to adjust to the unusual sensation and moving unaided may be difficult.

Pillows and back-rests. To reduce the risk of shearing tissue over the sacrum and heels the patient should be well supported when sitting up by using a back-rest and a careful arrangement of the pillows in arm-chair fashion. A foot-board placed either through the bed-cradle or supported by pillows at a suitable distance from the end of the bed against which to brace the feet will help to stop the patient from sliding down in the bed and will also help to prevent foot drop (see chapter 8). However busy she may be, the nurse should resist the temptation to try to pull the patient up the bed alone. Not only is this likely seriously to damage the skin and tissues over the patient's sacrum and heels, which latter are particularly vulnerable, but she also risks straining her own back.

Bed cradles should be used in the bed of any patient at risk of developing pressure sores, as the weight of the bed clothes can restrict the circulation and put undue pressure on the heels. The patient may need a small blanket around the feet to keep them warm.

Foam. Wedge-shaped foam pads, called *Lennards pads*, placed under the patient's legs are used to keep the heels clear of the bed without putting pressure on the calves. Heels can also be protected by *plastic foam or sheepskin 'socks'*.

(iii) Keeping the patient dry. To reduce the risk of sores it is obviously important to keep the skin dry. Ideally, incontinent patients should have their pads or sheets changed as soon as they become wet but this is not always possible where there is continual dribbling of urine. When a patient is wet, the area should be washed with soap and water and dried carefully. Powder is of doubtful value because it cakes in the skin folds and can cause sores, although it is pleasant for the patient to have a light dusting after a bath. Obese patients, who sweat profusely also need to have their skin washed and dried frequently. Silicone creams and sprays provide a waterproof barrier and will help to protect the skin of incontinent patients.

(iv) Skin applications. The nurse will probably encounter a diversity of opinions as to what should be applied to the skin to prevent pressure sores, and the practice varies from ward to ward. She must eventually decide for herself what is the most effective treatment from her experience of different methods and from her reading of research findings in the nursing journals. Soap and water are important for keeping the pressure areas clean, particularly the sacrum and buttocks. Either cream or powder (but never both) is used to prevent friction when massaging the pressure areas, but oil and cream applied excessively will make the skin soggy, and spirit dries the natural oils. Moisturising creams and those containing zinc, or talcum powder used sparingly, are probably the most useful.

(v) Massaging the pressure areas. The purpose of massaging the areas subjected to pressure is to stimulate a stagnant circulation. Massaging does not mean a vigorous rub with a handful of cream, which will increase the risk of the skin breaking, but a purposeful, circular motion, using the palm of the hand, gently moving the skin and subcutaneous tissues over the bony prominence beneath. After turning, it is those areas on which the patient *has been lying* where pressure has caused the circulation to stagnate, which should be treated.

(c) The general prevention of pressure sores

Nutrition. Patients who eat a well-balanced diet containing plenty of protein and vitamin C are unlikely to develop pressure sores. Where pressure sores have developed, or in the case of very debilitated patients, high-protein additives to the diet (Complan, Casilan, extra milk) will provide the essential amino-acids to rebuild the body's tissues. If the patient is extremely anaemic and has an extensive deep pressure sore a blood transfusion may be given (see Chapter 4) to speed the healing process, and its effect can be dramatic.

Mobility. Apart from any considerations of rehabilitation, the fact that movement inhibits the development of sores will be a great incentive to encourage patients to move themselves, by however little. All patients should be encouraged to wriggle their toes and move their feet in bed and when sitting in a chair, and patients sitting for long in chairs should have their feet on footstools to prevent oedema.

The treatment of pressure sores

When a pressure sore has developed the principles of treatment are:

> to relieve the pressure;
> to keep the area clean, dry and free from infection; and
> to ensure the patient has a nutritious diet.

Superficial sores. Small areas of broken skin and superficial sores should be cleaned with a mild antiseptic and covered by a dry dressing fixed with the minimum amount of a non-allergic adhesive tape. If it can be arranged, exposing the area to air or sunlight for short periods will encourage healing. A tiny break in the skin may be treated with a dab of tincture of benzoin compound applied with a sterile swab-stick; this will effectively seal the broken area and make a larger dressing unnecessary. (The patient should be warned that the tincture of benzoin will sting when applied.)

Deep sores. The treatment of a deep, necrotic sore is not such a hopeless task as it may at first seem. The dead tissue must be removed under the direction of the doctor, usually by cutting it away (débridement) with scissors. The raw area is then cleaned with eusol and packed with a dressing soaked in half-strength eusol until it is clean, which may take several weeks and will require frequent renewal of the packing.

Deep sores are often infected or prone to infection: in the former case a swab of the infected exudate will be sent for culture and testing for sensitivity, and an appropriate antibiotic ordered; in the latter a broad-spectrum antibiotic, such as penicillin with streptomycin, may be prescribed prophylactically.

When the granulation begins to occur care must be taken that any cavity undermining the skin is lightly packed to prevent the superficial layers healing over and leaving pockets of unhealed, infected tissue beneath. A variety of substances has been used for packing deep sores to encourage granulation including paraffin-impregnated gauze, cod-liver-oil ointment, and even honey. Sometimes the area of a deep sore will be skin-grafted. Ultra-violet light treatment may be given two or three times a week by the physiotherapist.

One of the more effective ways of cleaning a deep pressure sore, once the patient has become mobile, is to place her in a warm bath to which salt has been added. Not only will the area be cleaned but the patient will feel fresher. Because a healed pressure area never has as good a blood supply as the surrounding healthy tissue, great care must be taken to prevent it breaking down again.

A deep, necrotic pressure sore is generally less painful than a superficial sore because fewer nerve endings are exposed; but some patients may be acutely conscious of the large, raw area on their back which needs continual attention. Their distress may be severe enough to be a contributory cause of depression, which should be appreciated by the ward staff, as such sores may take months to heal. Other patients are surprisingly unaware of their sores although the smell of the exudate can be unpleasant and may be neutralised by a deodorant or air freshener, used either directly on the dressing or unobtrusively beside the bed.

2. The management of the incontinent patient

The reasons for urinary incontinence have been discussed in

Chapter 4 but the management of the incontinent patient is of particular importance in geriatric care. Incontinence is a major reason for the failure of successful rehabilitation because however mobile or independent such patients may be incontinence can prevent them from going home or even being admitted to certain old people's homes.

Most patients, unless they are severely depressed or demented, are embarrassed by their incontinence and will go to great lengths to disguise it. Few people are wilfully incontinent, although occasionally a patient will become incontinent in order to avoid being sent home or just to attract attention.

1. *Retraining the incontinent patient*

It is obviously important to distinguish between the patient whose mental impairment is so severe that, in the absence of conscious control, the emptying of the bladder becomes a reflex action, the patient who constantly dribbles urine as a result of damage to the urethral sphincter muscle and the patient who is incontinent but retains some bladder control and will therefore be amenable to retraining.

Investigations. Every incontinent patient should have a mid-stream specimen of urine tested for micro-organisms and for sugar (see Diabetes, p. 49). A rectal examination will show whether impacted faeces are disturbing normal functioning of the sphincters, and in male patients whether the prostate gland is enlarged. X-rays of the bladder will show the presence of bladder calculi, while a cystometrogram will measure the pressure within and the capacity of the bladder before its muscle wall begins to contract and the urethral sphincter relaxes.

Establishing a routine. Patients who are incontinent during the acute phase of an illness while they are confused, or who are incontinent because a urinary infection has caused frequency, will usually regain continence as their physical health improves. The patients needing most help are those whose incontinence is due to cerebral damage following a stroke or to inertia which is the result of depression or other emotional factors. Any patient who has recently had an indwelling catheter removed may also need help.

Incontinent patients need to be retrained to respond to the sensation of a full bladder. They will need to be offered a commode or, when mobile, help to walk to the lavatory, at two-hourly intervals during the day and at three-hourly intervals at night. Patients should not be asked if they want 'to pass water' as they will usually say they do not. If confined to bed the commode should be brought to them at regular times and, with curtains drawn round the bed, they should be asked to try to pass some water; if mobile they should be told that it is now time for them to be helped to the lavatory. It is essential for successful retraining to continue the régime at night, preferably by allowing patients to get out of bed to use the commode, for many elderly people find great difficulty in using a bedpan. The commode should be offered, even to a patient who has been incontinent.

A chart should be kept for each patient on which are recorded the time the commode was offered, whether or not urine was passed and whether the patient was incontinent; the same chart can be used to record bowel motions. The chart will give a good idea of the effectiveness of the retraining régime and the pattern of the patient's incontinence – whether more often incontinent at night, or in the morning after diuretics have been given – and it will also make sure that there is continuity between one shift of nurses and the next.

Patients should never be rebuked for being incontinent, however irritating it may be for those who care for them, nor should the nursing staff expect patients to remain continent if their request for a bedpan is ignored. Chapter 4 describes how elderly people suffer from precipitancy and frequency and this will be worse for those who have diuretics.

Patients cannot always be expected to retain urine until the next bedpan round and should be encouraged to think that they can ask for help whenever they feel the need. It is obviously in the best interests of both patients and staff that they should quickly become mobile enough to take themselves to the lavatory.

Fluid intake. Each patient should be encouraged to drink plenty of a variety of fluids (see section on Diets, p. 116), because highly concentrated urine will irritate the bladder and cause frequency. Some patients may find that their nocturnal incontinence improves if they do not drink after 5 p.m. but they should not allow themselves to become thirsty. Alcohol has a diuretic effect and its part in causing nocturnal incontinence must be weighed against its effectiveness as a mild sedative.

Drugs which disturb the action of the autonomic nervous system, such as probanthaline and atropine, may help to increase the bladder's capacity by relaxing the muscles of the bladder wall and inhibiting relaxation of the involuntary sphincter. These drugs can also cause drying of the saliva which will lead to sores developing in the mouth unless regular mouth care is given. Sedatives should be avoided wherever possible because they increase the likelihood of the patient being incontinent (see Sleep, p. 89).

As the patient becomes more continent so the interval between giving the commode or assistance to the lavatory can be increased, but even so, those patients who achieve continence will still need to be reminded to go to the lavatory. The need for continence in the rehabilitation wards is obvious and no nurse should resent the extra effort involved in ensuring patients use the commode or lavatory regularly.

The situation is different, however, in the long stay wards, where the patients are less mobile and more confused and the problems of taking them to the lavatory regularly are great. The effort may not seem worth while anyway if the patient continues to be incontinent; nevertheless, some patients do respond to this regular retraining and it is well worth persisting with those who are the most alert and mobile. The lingering smell of urine is evocative of the old, passive attitude to the nursing of elderly people and can help to create a very dismal impression of institutional care.

2. *Aids for incontinent patients*

There are a variety of aids to help people who are permanently incontinent to cope with it without resorting to catheterisation.
For men. The penile clamp is a simple device, particularly suitable for men who suffer from dribbling of urine following a prostatectomy, but the old person must be sufficiently alert

to cope with it. There is a variety of rubber and plastic urinals which are fitted to the penis by means of a condom or funnel inlet. During the day the urinal or drainage bag is strapped to the patient's leg but leakage at night is a common problem; such urinals also need a certain amount of co-operation from the patient.

In hospital, or even at home, an ordinary plastic urine bottle placed in position may be sufficient for the unconscious or chairbound patient who does not move very much. In an emergency, a simple device can be made using a contraceptive sheath, strapped to the penis by non-allergic tape, with a plastic connection passed through the teat end and attached to a length of tubing and a drainage bag.

For women. Some fitted urinals have been designed for women but these are not generally very effective, although research is being undertaken to develop a more reliable and comfortable one.

For the long-stay patient, a special chair with hole in the seat, under which slides a female urinal, may be helpful. However most incontinent patients will be nursed on plastic backed pads with a thick wadding and a special covering that keeps the surface of the pad dry. These are effective if changed frequently so that they do not become saturated. Patients who are relatively mobile should be fitted with pads and plastic pants (available in a variety of designs, some with a front-opening flap). The nurse should remember that disposable pads and other aids – incontinence tissues, plastic drawsheets, etc – are extremely expensive and create disposal problems so should be used as economically as possible.

3. *Catheterisation*

Temporary incontinence during an acute toxic confusional state or during the period of unconsciousness following a stroke is not an indication for catheterisation. The problems caused by catheterisation – increased risk of infection and damage to the sphincters – outweigh the problems of temporary incontinence when extra attention will be needed to ensure that the patient's sheet or pad is changed regularly and the skin of the buttocks and thighs is kept dry.

The chief indication of the need for an indwelling catheter occurs when the patient is incontinent and has a deep and extensive pressure sore, which will take very much longer to heal if the area is frequently wet. Once the sore is healing well and when the patient's physical condition has improved the catheter can be removed and a re-training régime started. For a period before the catheter is removed it should be clamped off and released for ten minutes every four hours in order to restore the muscle tone of the bladder wall.

Severely demented patients who have no control over their bladder may need to be catheterised but it depends on their degree of mobility and how liable they are to develop a pressure sore (see p. 103). If, despite mental impairment, they are mobile and physically well it may be possible to keep them relatively dry during the day with regular trips to the lavatory, while accepting that some incontinence is inevitable at night.

Care of the patient with an indwelling catheter. Geriatric patients are less able to tolerate an indwelling catheter than younger patients, and the confused, restless patient, in particular, may pull at it and cause trauma to the bladder neck with resulting haematuria. To prevent this the catheter should be firmly strapped to the patient's thigh with adhesive tape. If the patient is incontinent of faeces the catheter is likely to become soiled and, in order to prevent infection, it is particularly important that it should be cleaned meticulously every day or as soon as it becomes soiled, using an aseptic technique, with an antiseptic solution and cleaning *away* from the urethral orifice, using no swab more than once before discarding it.

A plastic, self-retaining catheter with a balloon (Gibbon or Foley) will need to be changed every two weeks and it is usual for the doctor to order a bladder washout with a mild antiseptic or saline solution whenever the catheter is changed. Patients with an indwelling catheter should be encouraged to drink plenty of fluids, and for the first few weeks of catheterisation their urinary output should be measured and recorded.

Occasionally a patient or the relatives can manage to cope with an indwelling catheter which is spiggotted off during the day and drained at intervals. At night it can be attached to a drainage tube and bag and fastened to the bed side rail.

3. Mouth care

Old people who are unable to chew their food easily because they have neither teeth nor dentures or whose dentures fit badly, will eat little, not enjoy their food and will be likely to suffer from indigestion.

Care of the teeth and dentures

The majority of elderly people have full or partial dentures. Many of the very elderly use them only for show because they were fitted so long ago that their gums have shrunk and the dentures now fit badly. Some old people manage to chew meat and fruit quite adequately with their gums and there is no reason why they should have new dentures unless they particularly want them. However, the majority of old people without adequate dentures limit themselves to soft, sloppy foods and would benefit considerably from a new set.

Hospital is a convenient place for the fitting of dentures, as most geriatric departments have a dentist who attends regularly, so obviating the need for patients to make several visits to a distant surgery, which may discourage them. As it takes a little time to get used to new dentures, the nurse must encourage her patients to wear them and not remove them at meal times. Patients who have had a cerebral vascular accident which has affected their facial muscles may find difficulty in keeping their dentures in place. They should be encouraged to wear them for short periods to prevent their gums from shrinking; the dentist may be able to adjust them to fit better.

Dentures should be cleaned at least once a day and stored in one of the special cleansing solutions at night. A mouth wash will help to remove debris stuck to the gums and will freshen the mouth.

Patients with some of their own teeth remaining may need dental treatment. Some may never have been to the dentist and are quite unable to chew adequately with the few stumps or carious teeth that remain. It will need a skilful nurse to persuade such a patient to be treated and it may help if the initial dental examination is done in the ward in familiar surroundings.

The nurse who admits any patient should note the state of the teeth and whether or not dentures are worn.

General mouth care

Elderly patients need special attention to their mouths. Many are unable to clean their own teeth properly or do not clean their dentures. Many regularly cough up thick sputum, and digestive disturbances or chronic constipation can cause furring of the tongue and an unpleasant taste in the mouth; these patients should be encouraged to clean their teeth and dentures, and they should also be given a mouth wash twice a day and – it cannot be stressed enough – encouraged to drink plenty of fluids. Fresh fruit also helps to cleanse the mouth. Well-chewed food stimulates the production of saliva which helps to keep the mouth clean and makes the food taste better; this stimulates the appetite which, in turn, increases the secretion of gastric juices, thereby improving digestion.

Drugs that increase the capacity of the bladder (such as probanthiline) may cause the saliva in the mouth to dry up, which increases the risk of the mouth becoming sore; particular attention should be paid to the mouth-care of patients on these drugs. Patients who are unconscious, semi-conscious and very ill need regular mouth toilet. Their mouths should be cleaned four times a day, or more often if necessary, with pledgets of cotton wool, changed frequently, firmly held in clip forceps and dipped in glycothymoline mouth wash or glycerine and borax. All parts of the mouth are cleaned in a systematic way, and afterwards dry and cracked lips may be lubricated with a little petroleum jelly.

4. The diet of the elderly patient

An adequate diet is not only an important part of any patient's treatment but mealtimes are a major focus of interest in the patient's day. The junior nurse has little control over the food sent from the kitchen for patients' meals, but by preparing the patients so that they are able to enjoy their food and by serving it in an attractive way, she has considerable control over what actually is eaten.

Constituents of an adequate diet. Old people have as much need for protein to replace the worn-out tissue cells as have younger persons, but require less carbohydrate. A fairly active, retired man requires about 2,300 calories a day and a woman needs about 2,100, reducing with age and increasing immobility.

Iron, found in red meat, liver, eggs and green vegetables, is needed to maintain the body's stores and for the manufacture of red blood corpuscles which continue to be replaced until death. *Calcium*, found in milk, cheese, fish and meat is important in the diet of elderly people because a deficiency of calcium is thought to be a contributory cause of osteoporosis. *Vitamin C*, found in fresh fruit and vegetables, is the vitamin most likely to be deficient in an old person's diet.

Roughage is particularly important in the diet of the elderly who have a tendency to constipation which may be partly due to a slower peristaltic action, as it forms the bulk of the stool and makes it easier to pass. Roughage is found in unrefined cereals, e g brown flour, whole wheat breakfast cereals, bran, fresh fruit, salads and vegetables. Two tablespoons of bran taken daily could prevent the misery and discomfort of chronic constipation and the nurse can play a part in trying to encourage this habit.

Fluids. Many old people restrict the amount they drink to reduce their need to go to the lavatory, which is dangerous because they may take insufficient fluids to flush through the waste products of metabolism, such as urea (see Chapter 2). Concentrated, and possibly subsequently infected urine irritates the bladder causing frequency and precipitancy. If the body is short of water, more fluid will be drawn from the faecal waste in the large bowel, leaving the stool hard and dry and increasing constipation. In severe cases the patient may become dehydrated.

Malnutrition. The majority of old people in Britain have a reasonable diet, but those living alone and the lonely, especially widowers, and the disabled are the most likely to have an inadequate diet. Meals on Wheels and Luncheon

Clubs (see Chapter 8) have helped to alleviate this problem, for old people can get a substantial part of their weekly protein and iron needs from two or three meals supplied in this way.

Obesity. The main problem of malnutrition among the elderly is overfeeding, which causes obesity. Overweight people are seriously handicapped, with increased risk of heart failure, hypertension, osteo-arthritis, diabetes and chest disease. Obesity may have been a life-long problem. 'I have always been of a big build' or 'it runs in the family', or it may have developed with old age as the old person persists, despite decreasing activity, with a diet which is high in carbohydrates. Old people with a low income which leaves little to spend on food will tend to buy the cheaper foods, bread, potatoes, cereals, sugar and biscuits, all of which are particularly high in carbohydrates. This diet will satisfy them and if they do not understand the importance of a balanced diet will tend to buy these foods rather than the more expensive meat and fish, or items that are more difficult to prepare such as fruit and vegetables.

It is an extremely difficult task to persuade old people to lose weight and there seems little point in demanding a very strict diet if their last years are going to be made miserable. However, a nurse can use her good influence with the obese patient by pointing out the dangers of being overweight and by stressing which foods cause the weight problem. She may also be able to persuade the old person to stop eating sweets, sweet biscuits and jam and to reduce her consumption of bread and potatoes.

Diet in hospital. The geriatric ward is not the ideal place to reform an elderly person's diet. The catering department should offer a choice of diet so the patient may be encouraged to try something different. Fresh fruit brought in for the patient is a good alternative to the ubiquitous milk pudding or jelly but it will so often be left to deteriorate in the bowl unless the nurse takes trouble to prepare it. Relatives and friends are often willing to provide extras and will usually welcome suggestions about what to bring; some will go as far as to bring in prepared meals, and if the patient requests a jar of jellied eels it will be just as nourishing as a lamb chop – and enjoyed much more!

Fluid balance. Unless it is necessary for medical reasons to restrict their fluid intake, elderly patients need to drink between 1500 and 2000 ml a day; most elderly people need almost continual encouragement to drink more. Fruit squashes are ideal for making water palatable for patients unaccustomed to drinking anything but tea, and the medicine round provides a good opportunity to persuade a reluctant patient to drink another glassful. Many elderly people find the conventional hospital tumbler too heavy and wide to handle easily and are discouraged, but there is a variety of light plastic beakers which are easier to manage. Feeding cups and flexible straws are other aids for the more helpless patients. Every patient, whether in bed or sitting up at the table in the day room, should always have a drink within reach.

Ale and stout are very acceptable forms of fluid in the geriatric ward and a source of vitamin B. Many patients are delighted to find they are medicinal! No alcohol should be given to a patient without consulting a senior nurse, as the effect of some drugs is enhanced by alcohol, and as alcohol is also a diuretic, some patients with a restricted bladder capacity may find that drinking beer causes frequency.

It is often difficult to keep an accurate fluid balance chart for elderly patients, and rarely necessary in geriatric care. The time and effort spent in maintaining a neat, but probably not very accurate, chart of intake and output will detract from the time needed to ensure that the patient drinks sufficient fluid. It is the duty of every nurse to persuade patients to drink as much as possible and the importance of this should be explained to ward orderlies and volunteers who distribute drinks, so that they in turn can encourage patients to have their drinks rather than leave them untouched.

Occasionally, however, if a patient is severely ill in cardiac or renal failure, is having a blood transfusion or intravenous fluids, has been admitted severely dehydrated, or is passing urine inadequately, it will be necessary to maintain a careful fluid balance chart.

Serving foods and feeding patients

Serving food. Patients should be prepared for their meal before it is brought to them. Those in bed should be sitting up, well supported by pillows with the bed table drawn up to them, and those who are out of bed should be encouraged to sit at the communal dining table; but when they are not well enough to do this, an individual table should be drawn up over their knees, so that they can reach their food comfortably. There is a variety of bibs available for adults but as bibs have an unfortunate association with babies elderly people may feel insulted by wearing them. A gaily-coloured, sleeveless cotton smock that opens down the back looks attractive, and will protect the patient's clothes, not only from food, but also from newsprint and ballpoint ink. Patients should be wearing their dentures, and their hands may need to be washed.

Many elderly people have conservative ideas about food but it is possible to vary their diet by offering something they would nor normally choose. Those who choose milk pudding from habit will probably eat stewed fruit with custard if this is served instead. Food should be served hot if it is meant to be hot, on a warmed plate, and similarly cold food should be served cold. Patients not feeling well will find a large portion unappetising and it is better to serve a small amount which looks pleasant and then ask if they would like more. For those patients who need to have their food cut up, it is more tactful to do this before taking the plate to them.

Feeding aids. Patients should feed themselves whenever possible. They may need special cutlery with extra wide handles or with a spoon that swivels within a solid handle, and the occupational therapist will advise on this. A cereal bowl may be more suitable for the main course than a dinner plate and few elderly patients can manage to eat a boiled egg from its shell but if it is turned out into a warmed bowl they will be quite independent. Acute and continuous observation by all the staff is necessary to ensure that patients can manage, and it is surprising how a simple re-arrangement such as the offer of a spoon and fork instead of a knife and fork, can make a patient independent and able to enjoy her food at her own speed.

Feeding patients

Feeding is a skill that is not easy to acquire. To make the meal acceptable the nurse must be prepared to spend as much time over feeding a patient as the patient herself would normally take. It is here that relatives and volunteers are invaluable, for they have the time to sit and talk while they are feeding the patient and thus make the mealtime the interesting social event it should be.

Great care must be taken when feeding and giving drinks to patients whose swallowing mechanism is affected, as it may be after a pseudo-bulbar palsy or certain cerebro-vascular accidents (see Chapter 4). Food should not be too sloppy and it should be given slowly, with careful observation of how well the patient is swallowing. The danger is that patients may choke and inhale food into their trachea. No inexperienced person should give food or drinks to such patients, and it is advisable to keep an electric suction machine near them so that should they choke the food can be aspirated from the back of the throat. In extreme cases, it may be necessary to pass a naso-gastric tube.

Feeding by naso-gastric tube. The use of a naso-gastric tube for feeding elderly patients should be avoided if at all possible, because older people find the passing of the tube particularly distressing and do not tolerate it well, and a confused patient is likely to pull it out as soon as it is passed.

The only indications for feeding by naso-gastric tube are (*a*) when the swallowing mechanism is affected (see above), or (*b*) when a patient has been unconscious for more than 24-48 hours, as after a cerebral haemorrhage. A patient suffering from an acute toxic confusional state can usually be persuaded to drink some fluid, but if severely dehydrated, an intravenous infusion is usually considered more suitable.

Particular care must be taken when passing a tube into the stomach of an elderly patient who has suffered a stroke because partial paralysis of the pharyngeal muscles will increase the risk of the tube passing into the trachea. The stomach contents should be aspirated and tested with litmus paper (which should produce an acid reaction if the tube is correctly sited) before any nourishment is given through the tube. The tube should be re-checked before each feed to ensure that it has remained in the stomach and is not coiled up in the back of the throat. A conscious patient will cough and react strongly if a gastric tube is passed into the respiratory tract in error, but as the swallowing and coughing reflexes of the unconscious or semi-conscious patient are absent, or diminished, the nurse must be on the alert for any change in the patient's colour, which will indicate respiratory obstruction, and immediately remove the tube.

5. The administration of drugs

A geriatric patient may be prescribed as many as seven or eight different medications a day, and not only must the nurse check that what she is giving tallies with the prescription, and is recorded carefully, but she must make sure that each patient does in fact take all the prescribed medicines. Medicines or tablets must never be left on a locker for the patient to take later, however well orientated and sensible the person may be; many elderly people are suspicious of medicines and will go to great lengths to avoid taking them, or they may genuinely forget. While the nurse should always stay by the patient to make sure the medicines are swallowed, she need not do this obtrusively; old people need time to swallow tablets and will appreciate a glass of water or fruit drink with which to wash them down.

The larger tablets and capsules are particularly difficult for elderly patients to swallow. Some tablets can be crushed between two metal spoons and the powder given in a small medicine glass with some water, dry on a spoon or even wrapped in a piece of bread, but crushing may be unsuitable if the tablets or capsules are compounded in such a way as to reduce irritation to the gastric mucosa or to delay absorption of the drug. If the tablets are unsuitable for crushing or the patient cannot take them crushed, it may be possible for the pharmacist to make up the drug as a suspension; as with most medicines, it is important that such a suspension be well shaken before the dose is measured. Any patient continually refusing to take a drug, or who spits it back must be reported to the ward sister who will seek the doctor's instructions; the drug may then be discontinued or given in some other form.

All medicines, whether liquid or tablets and including aperients, should be recorded as soon as they have been taken. Most elderly patients are unlikely to remember what they have had and it is obviously necessary for the doctor to know exactly what has been given in order to assess the effectiveness of the treatment. While this must be the routine procedure for any ward, the number and variety of drugs given to patients in geriatric wards is on a scale not usually seen elsewhere so particular care must be taken.

Although some old people are suspicious of taking medicines, many others set great store by their tablets and will come into hospital with a large selection which have been prescribed or bought over the counter for many years past. As the doctor must know what the patient has been taking before admission, the admitting nurse is responsible for finding out what medicines the patient has brought into hospital and for removing these. This can be done tactfully: 'The doctor will want to know what you have been taking, Mrs G.; may I take these to show him? He may not want you to have these now as they will not mix well with what he is going to prescribe for you.' Patients may have spent a lot of money on patent medicines which they feel are helpful and if the doctor agrees that taking them can do no harm, these should be returned when they go home. Hospital staff sometimes find it difficult to realise that patients have survived for many years without their help, very often treating minor complaints by self-medication and that they may have more trust in a patent medicine taken for years than in some new tablets, supplied by a doctor they have known for only a few weeks. In any case, all patients should be given a simple explanation of what each medicine or tablet is for so that they can appreciate the need to take them.

6. Accidents in the ward

Elderly people, because of their unsteadiness, poor sight and deafness are particularly at risk of injury from accidents both inside and outside hospital. In hospital, a few accidents will be inevitable when patients are encouraged to be as active and independent as possible. The common accidents are falls, either from a standing position or from bed, burns from hot food and liquids, radiators and fires, and cuts and bruises from knocks against furniture.

Prevention of accidents. Nurses have a particular responsibility for ensuring that as far as possible, accidents are anticipated and prevented. Patients most likely to fall are the frail, the hemiplegic and the confused and they must be given the correct aids or sufficient support to help them. A patient who stands up incorrectly, uses a walking frame wrongly or tries to get from bed to chair without enough support is risking a fall and should be taught how to execute these movements safely (see Chapter 8). Wet and highly polished floors are dangerous, so that spills should be mopped up at once and the ward domestic staff discouraged from using too much polish or water when cleaning the floors. Trailing chair blankets and small pieces of furniture, like footstools, are particular hazards.

Falls from bed are not necessarily prevented by the use of cot-sides (see Chapter 6). Patients likely to climb out of bed when confused should be in beds which can be under continual observation by the nursing staff, and their movements should be anticipated.

Burns can be prevented by making sure that fires and radiators are protected by guards and by not allowing those patients likely to spill food or drink, anything very hot; suitable utensils, like feeding cups and adapted spoons can help to prevent spills. Knocks against furniture can be avoided by ensuring that patients have suitable aids to help them and that chairs, trolleys, etc. are not left in passageways, to be a hazard for those patients with poor eyesight.

Immediate treatment. No accident, however minor should be ignored. Old people's bones fracture with very little trauma and the shock following a burn may be out of all proportion to the severity of the burn. Patients who are obviously seriously injured after a fall, should be covered with a blanket and not moved; otherwise it is usually safe to help them to a chair or lift them into bed. Any witness of a fall may be able to give some clue to the cause of it – a temporary hypoxia of the brain, when the patient would appear to collapse, or a real accident, when the patient trips or slips – and a clear account will help the doctor assess likely injuries.

Burns and scalds should be treated with particular care to prevent further damage to the skin and infection, as they may take a long time to heal, especially those on the shins and feet. The burnt area should be covered with a sterile dressing pad and a doctor called to examine it as soon as possible.

Reporting accidents. Hospital procedure for reporting accidents varies but any patient who suffers an injury in the ward or any part of the hospital, or is involved in an accident in any way, must have the incident recorded. A doctor should examine the patient as soon as possible after an accident and treat any injuries. He should write an account of the accident, and of his examination and treatment of the patient, in the patient's notes and the nurse in charge should write her own account of what occurred in the nursing notes and fill in the details on the appropriate accident form provided by the hospital. Anything but a very minor accident should be reported to a senior nursing officer and the relatives must be told what has happened when they visit, or in serious cases, contacted by telephone and told.

It occasionally happens that the patient will die soon after an accident and if injury is thought to have been a contributory cause of death, the coroner at the inquest will require an account of the accident. A clear report of the incident in the patient's notes and the nursing notes may make it unnecessary for a witness to attend and will help to avoid unpleasant recriminations from relatives.

7. Lifting and moving the patient and heavy equipment

As so much lifting of both patients and equipment is done in geriatric wards, the nurse must train herself automatically to lift correctly; many nurses have seriously damaged their backs by lifting a patient or a heavy piece of equipment, probably when they were in a hurry. Serious back injury can cause severe pain and be very incapacitating, even to the extent of costing the nurse her job. A quite minor back strain may necessitate weeks of sick leave and an increased risk of further injury.

Rules for lifting
(1) Do not try to lift anything that is obviously too heavy, no matter how short-staffed the ward may be.
(2) Do not lift things to an unnecessary height. Wheel a bed out of the way rather than try to lift a chair over it.
(3) Avoid bending forward initially more than is necessary, e g raise an adjustable bed to a convenient height. When preparing to lift and during lifting, keep the back straight, bend the knees slightly and use the muscles of the legs, buttocks, arms and shoulders to take the strain.
(4) Keep the object to be lifted as close to the body as possible: lifting at arms' length is inefficient and makes it more difficult to keep a straight back.

Lifting and turning the patient
The Australian or shoulder lift. This lift is the most efficient way to move patients up the bed and in most cases to lift them from the bed to a chair and back again. The bed should be adjusted to the height of a normal hospital bed to reduce the distance the nurses have to bend.
(1) Two nurses face each other on either side of the patient, standing with their feet about eighteen inches apart.
(2) The patient must be sitting leaning forward. (If help is required to sit forward, the nurses pass their arms under the patient's axillae and gently incline her forward with their hands on her scapulae and not gripping her upper arms.)
(3) As the patient leans forward, the nurses turn their bodies toward the top of the bed, bend their knees and slide their shoulders into the patient's armpits, allowing the patient's arms to rest along their backs.
(4) They grip each other's inside wrist or hand beneath the patient's thighs. Their other hand can be braced against the bedhead or on to the mattress.
(5) At a given word, each nurse presses her shoulder into the patient's axilla; by straightening her knees and keeping her

back straight, the leverage of each nurse's shoulder lifts the patient, her back foot taking the weight. (As the patient is lifted clear of the bed, a third nurse can straighten the sheet, change the pad or slip in a bed pan.)

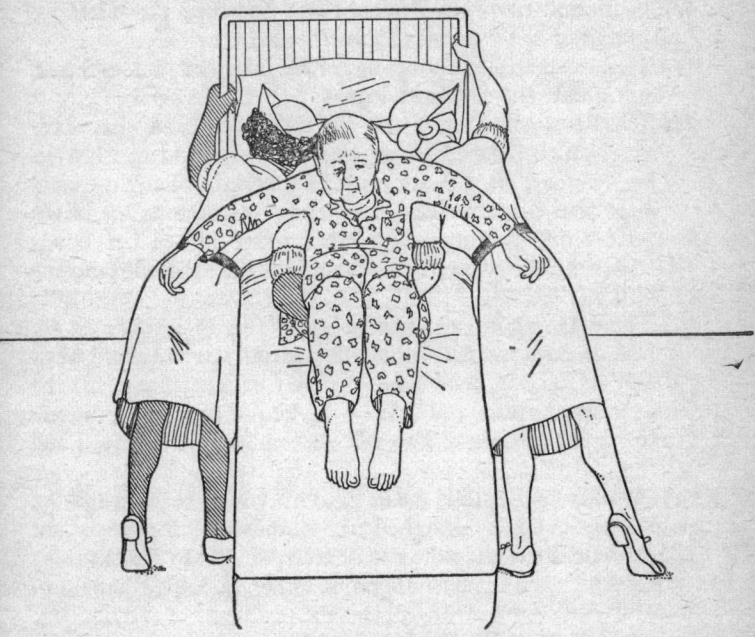

FIG. 2 The Australian Lift

(6) By transferring the weight from their back to their front foot, the nurses can move the patient up the bed and gently lower her into the new position. If no third person is available to help and the patient is not too heavy, the nurses lifting can hold the patient clear of the bed and with their free hand straighten the sheet, etc. It is important to lift well clear of the bed so that there is no risk of the patient being dragged over the sheet. Whenever possible the patient can help to take some of the weight by pulling on the rope or chain above the bed.

Turning a patient in bed. The patient who is nursed in a semi-prone or lateral position will need to be turned frequently. Before turning a patient, all but one of the pillows should be removed, and the blankets turned down leaving a sheet or washable blanket to cover the patient; the bed cradle is removed, and the urine drainage bag and tube passed across and attached to the other side of the bed.

(1) Two nurses stand one on either side of the bed and straighten the patient's legs.
(2) The nurse standing at the patient's back places her forearms on the patient's shoulders and hips and gently rolls her onto her back. Care must be taken to maintain a clear airway in an unconscious patient by continuous use of the semi-prone position. The other nurse places her hands under the hips and shoulders and rolls the patient onto the opposite side.
(3) The patient's hip and knee joints of the uppermost leg are flexed. Both nurses link hands beneath the patient's waist and thighs and, while keeping their backs straight, lift the buttocks towards the side of the bed in order to maintain the lateral position. The pillows can then be replaced and the bed remade.

A variety of hoists is available with which to help lift the patient out of bed or into the bath but most require the patient either to be lifted on to the seat or rolled on to the slings.

The advice of the physiotherapist can be valuable when nursing staff are confronted with specific problems of moving and lifting patients, and relatives will appreciate some expert guidance on how to lift and move a helpless old person at home.

For Further Reading

Agate, J. *Geriatrics for Nurses and Social Workers*. Heinemann, 1972

Edmondson, E. *Nursing the Incontinent Patient*. Butterworth, 1971

Norton, D., Mclaren, R. & Exton-Smith, A. N. *Geriatric Nursing Problems in Hospital*. Churchill-Livingstone, 1975

Stanton, B. R. *Meals for the Elderly*. King Edward's Hospital Fund for London, 1971

Physiotherapy Helps Nursing. Nursing Times Reprint, 1963

8. Rehabilitation

Rehabilitation and re-ablement are words commonly used by those involved in geriatric care and have a similar meaning which can be defined as 'the progressive treatment given to patients to enable them to

(a) achieve the maximum state of independence of which they are capable;
(b) cope with their individual needs of living, through the restoration of function and skills.'

Everyone who comes into contact with patients in hospital can contribute to their rehabilitation, from the doctor who treats an initial infection to the physiotherapist who plans a progression of exercises for them, from the junior nurse who helps them into and out of bed to the ward orderly who, by placing a cup of tea within reach, encourages them to feed themselves.

Early care

Rehabilitation begins immediately the patient is admitted to the ward. It is unlikely that complete bed rest will be ordered, and patients should be encouraged to do as much for themselves as they can. In the early stages of an acute illness, such as bronchitis, this may be no more than washing their own face or supporting the cup while they drink. Patients who are confined to bed must be lifted, turned, and positioned so that they are able to help themselves, being taught how this can be done to incur the least effort and avoid undue exhaustion. At meal times, their pillows must support them sitting upright, so that they can reach out to feed themselves. The locker must be within easy reach and moved to the other side of the bed as the patient is turned, a point that is often forgotten.

Passive exercises. Very weak or helpless patients, particularly following a stroke, may be unable to move their limbs and it is important that the muscles are not allowed to become wasted through disuse and the joints stiffened and contracted into a fixed position. If each limb is put through its full range of movements daily by the physiotherapist or nurse, not only will deformities be prevented but the blood supply to area will be improved by the exercise and the risk of pressure sores will be lessened. Those patients who are able to move their limbs should be encouraged to do this each time they are turned or washed, helped by the nurse supporting the weight of the limb.

As the acute phase of the illness passes, patients will be encouraged to do more for themselves and it will become easier to plan positive rehabilitation, which will depend on

(a) assessment of the patients' individual capabilities and needs,
(b) the attitude of patients and their relatives to self-help,
(c) a plan of treatment that involves the gradual withdrawal of support and nursing care so that the patients learn to be more independent.

Assessment of capability. The period spent in the assessment ward (see Chapter 5) will be used to plan the programme of rehabilitation. Some patients recover quickly from an acute illness and can be discharged home directly from the assessment ward with little formal rehabilitation but the majority will need longer to reach their maximum independence. Rehabilitation is the essence of the specialist care offered by the geriatric department and some patients are admitted solely to be rehabilitated.

The nursing staff make contact with patients during their first few days in the ward and they are in the best position to judge how far each patient is willing and able to help herself. Elderly people move slowly and cautiously in unfamiliar surroundings. They must be given time to perform simple tasks like washing their face and hands: while it may be quicker for the nursing staff to do it for them it is contrary to the aims of rehabilitation to deprive them of this opportunity to help themselves. Ward meetings can be used by the staff to discuss the capabilities of each patient and the amount of help each needs; thus: 'Mr A. would help himself more if he could get out of bed on the right-hand side, it's the side he is used to'; or 'Miss C. manages to dress very well as long as she has her clothes by her left hand.'

Later, as the physiotherapist undertakes more formal rehabilitation she will assess the degree to which each patient can tolerate exercise. One patient may tire quickly while another may lack the ability to concentrate for more than a short time so that it may be necessary to break down the sequence of exercises into a progression of simpler actions to maintain a steady improvement.

Assessment of the patient's needs. The aim of all rehabilitation programmes is to restore the patient to at least the degree of independence enjoyed before the illness that brought about admission to hospital. It is therefore important to have a full report of the patient's social situation and the help received from friends, relatives and the community services. Two patients whose degree of independence is quite different illustrates this point:

'Mrs J., a widow who lives alone and manages well with the help of a daughter who does her heavier shopping and housework, is admitted with acute bronchitis and anaemia. If she is to return to her home she must not only be independent of nursing care but also be able to cook simple meals, manage her pension and cope with tasks around the house such as lighting the fire and answering the door. At first she may have the help of visits from the home nurse, and a home help may be available, but for most of the day she will have to care for herself. It is obvious that she should not be allowed to become too dependent, either physically or emotionally, while she is in hospital'.

'Mr D., on the other hand, has lived with a devoted daughter for many years. She does all the shopping, cooking and housework. Following a fall he has been virtually bed-ridden and he is admitted specifically for rehabilitation. To relieve the pressure of care on his daughter he must, by the time he is discharged from hospital, be able to get in and out of bed unaided, walk short distances to a commode or lavatory, wash, dress and feed himself. It would be unreasonable to expect him to start cooking and housework but involvement in diversional activities may give him new interests and skills.'

Climbing stairs is, for some patients, a major obstacle to their returning home and any rehabilitation must include practising on the stairs. It is, of course, unnecessary to put patients who have no need to climb stairs through the strenuous and perhaps frightening experience of relearning this skill. (See Fig. 9).

The patient's attitude. Before any rehabilitation programme can be effective, the patient herself must want to get better. Some elderly people put up a great struggle before accepting admission and once in hospital they seem to lose any desire to get well again. It is a sad fact that many people still think of a geriatric ward as a place to which the old are sent to die. A patient believing this may say 'Don't make me do this, I only want to die'. This creates an extraordinarily difficult situation and the answer is not to brush aside such a comment with a breezy 'Of course you don't. Upsi-daisy!' which will only increase the patient's resentment towards any efforts to get her mobilised. The situation is best discussed with other members of the geriatric team so that a common approach can be made to such patients. Those who react like this may have led isolated, lonely lives and find it difficult to realise that people do care about the quality of the life they lead. If the ward staff can show their interest and care in them as people as well as in the progress they make towards helping themselves, they may learn to value their own efforts.

Admission to hospital may be a welcome break from the monotony of loneliness and the struggle to cope with shopping and cooking, or an escape from the hostile atmosphere of a relative's home. Unless such feelings are understood, encouraging patients to be independent may have little effect in the face of the realisation that the quicker the recovery the sooner will come discharge from the security of the hospital. It is not easy to change the social circumstances of a person (the possibilities are discussed in Chapter 9) and it is more helpful to accustom patients to the idea of going back to their old life with all the help that is available than to offer something which is unrealistic. Patients may be very worried that they will be sent home before they can cope and should be reassured that help will be provided.

Some patients see no reason why they should be 'made to get up' when they still feel unwell, as for example:

'Mrs T., who was admitted for investigations of urinary incontinence, thought herself more ill than she was. She was used to being cared for by a devoted and indulgent husband and she insisted that she was better resting in bed and that if she was made to get up she would not get dressed. Such a situation needed firm handling by the doctors and nurses, who explained that it would be more detrimental to her health to remain in bed.'

Reluctant patients may sometimes be persuaded to get dressed if they are reminded that it will please their relatives and that they themselves will feel better. Patients who resist all attempts at rehabilitation, either by refusing to co-operate or by appearing fearful of doing the simplest task are likely to be suffering from acute anxiety, depression or the mental state associated with arteriosclerotic dementia.

Relatives' attitudes. The close relatives of the patient should understand the purpose and importance of any rehabilitation programme. All too often, the relative responsible for caring for an elderly person is led to believe that the patient will be able to stay in hospital permanently. As can be seen now, this is not the purpose of a geriatric department and unless its rehabilitative function has been explained to the family it is understandable that some may be disconcerted to find their elderly relative being encouraged to get out of bed and get dressed when they had expected her to be nursed passively into oblivion.

The doctor and senior nurse are responsible for explaining to the relatives what is hoped will be the outcome of the patient's treatment, but it is, however, often the junior nurse, the one who is seen to be caring most for the patient, who appears to the anxious relative to be the more approachable. The nurse who is approached by a relative can arrange for her to see the nurse in charge. Once the purpose of the rehabilitation programme has been explained and the effects of it begin to show, many relatives will co-operate and appreciate the results. Some elderly people are over-indulged by devoted relatives, particularly daughters, who are then amazed to see how much a previously unco-operative person will do when persuaded.

Planning a rehabilitation programme

Different rehabilitation programmes can be planned for three categories of patient. They are:

(a) *For the patient, who, although physically able, has lost confidence* following a fall or an acute illness, or who has been immobile for a long time because of a debilitating illness such as anaemia or myxoedema.

The aim of the programme is: 1. to improve gradually the patient's ability to help herself with washing, dressing and walking, in the ward; 2. with the help of the physiotherapist, to restore confidence in walking, climbing stairs, etc; 3. to restore independence by practising, under the supervision of the occupational therapist, the functional activities of daily living – cooking, washing up, and running a house.

(b) *For the patient who is disabled* as the result of arthritis, Parkinson's disease, a fractured femur, etc.

The programme will be similar to that of the patient who is physically able but the physiotherapist may first have to correct faults of posture and walking before introducing specific exercises for improving the movement of a particular joint or limb. The occupational therapist can supply aids to help with dressing, cooking and housework.

(c) *For the patient who has had a stroke.* The programme in this case will be more specific and will depend upon the extent of the disabilities caused by the stroke. The purpose of rehabilitation will be to re-educate the affected limbs and to teach the patient to make full use of the rest of her body to compensate for the loss of function resulting from the stroke. Successful rehabilitation following a stroke can take a very long time and will continue after the patient has left hospital.

The rôle of the doctor

The doctor initiates and co-ordinates the rehabilitation programme for each patient and will require regular reports of the patient's progress from the nursing staff and therapists;

everyone concerned with the patient's rehabilitation will be able to contribute. He may prescribe analgesics for patients who find movements painful so that they are able to work more easily with the physiotherapist and take full advantage of the exercises. Analgesic drugs must be given at the correct time before the physiotherapy sessions.

The doctor will plan the discharge of the patients when he considers they are sufficiently independent and, with the senior nurse and the social worker, will keep the relatives informed of the patient's progress.

The rôle of the nurse

The nurse remains with the patients for most of the day and is responsible for helping them with the basic activities of getting in and out of bed, dressing and feeding. The nurse must remind herself whenever she is assisting patients that the aim of rehabilitation is to withdraw support gradually and to allow them to do as much as they are able for themselves, however slowly. The patient who comes to rely upon the nurse's help will take longer to become independent.

General rehabilitation

Each action undertaken by a patient should be broken down into simple movements and equipment should as far as possible simulate home conditions. For example, hospital beds are usually higher than those at home and must either be lowered or provided with a sturdy footstool. The patient should be encouraged to get in and out of the side she would use at home.

(a) **Getting out of bed.** The patient should be shown how to:
1. Roll to one side with knees bent by bringing one hand across the body and pulling on the side of the bed.
2. Using the upper hand, lever herself onto her elbow and into a sitting position. Swing her legs over the side of the bed and balance there supporting herself with both hands on the edge of the bed.
3. Slither along the edge of the bed to where the chair or commode has been placed parallel to and facing the head of the bed.
4. With the hand which is nearer the foot of the bed, reach

for the further arm of the chair, the other hand still on the edge of the bed.
5. Slide off the edge of the bed until the feet are flat on the ground and pivot through 90° to sit in the chair.

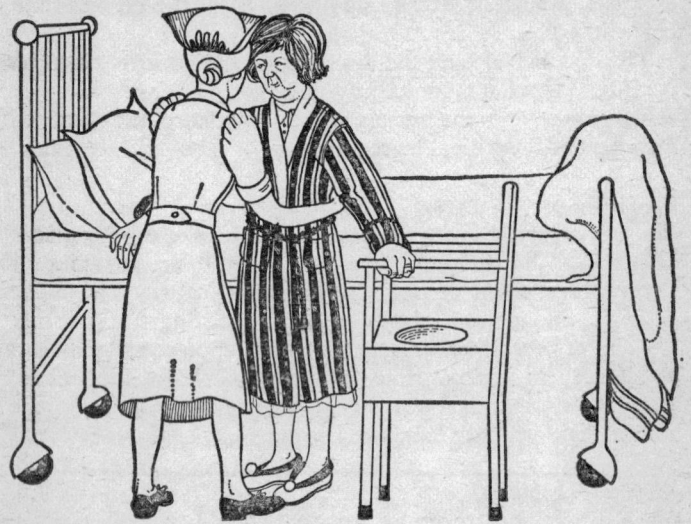

FIG. 3 Assisting the patient from her bed to the commode

The nurse can assist the patient into a sitting position by supporting the body from under the axillae while the patient levers herself onto one elbow. As the patient slides from the bed the nurse can give the maximum support by facing the patient and encircling her arms around the patient's waist, keeping her own back straight and pivoting with the patient. To prevent the patient's feet slipping as she slides onto them the nurse can place one of her own feet in fron of them.

Unless shown the simple ways of doing these everyday actions, the patient is likely to use unnecessary effort, turn awkwardly and lose her balance. A fall may cause loss of confidence and delay progress for some time, so careful instruction and preparation for each movement are important.
(b) Getting back into bed. The above process is reversed but the patient must remember that it is easier to turn through one

quarter of a circle than through three quarters. With the chair placed alongside the bed facing the bedhead, the patient should
(1) stand up using the arms of the chair for support (see (f) below;
(2) transfer the hand *nearest* the bed to the rail at the head of the bed;
(3) pivot backwards through 90° and ease the buttocks onto the edge of the bed; and
(4) press down with both hands placed on the edge of the bed and lever the body back into the centre of the bed and then swing the legs on to the bed.

If the bed is high a frail patient will find this manoeuvre difficult. A footstool or the seat of a chair on which to place the feet before lifting backwards can give additional leverage. A rope suspended from a support fitted over the bed on which the patient can pull to lift herself may also be necessary, but if it is the only means by which she can get into bed a similar device must be provided at home if independence is to be achieved.

(c) End of bed exercises. These simple exercises can be done in the ward as a prelude to walking. Ideally the patient should be sitting in a high armchair facing the rail at the end of the bed or a bar at a suitable height (about the level of the elbows when the patient is sitting). A board against the wheels of the bed will prevent the patient's feet from sliding forward, and when exercising, low-heeled walking shoes should be worn rather than slippers.

The patient practises pulling herself up out of the chair by holding on to the bar until standing upright with feet slightly apart, facing forwards with knees straight, then lowers herself back into the chair. At first two nurses can help with the initial leverage by supporting the patient under the axillae. Once able to stand and sit easily the patient can take a step or two to either side still holding on to the bar.

A simple way to transfer a heavy patient from a chair to a wheelchair or commode is for the patient to stand up using the rail while one chair is substituted for the other and then to lower herself into the sitting position.

These exercises help to give the patient confidence and to

regain a sense of balance, strengthen arm and leg muscles, improve the circulation to buttocks and thighs and relieve pressure on the sacrum.

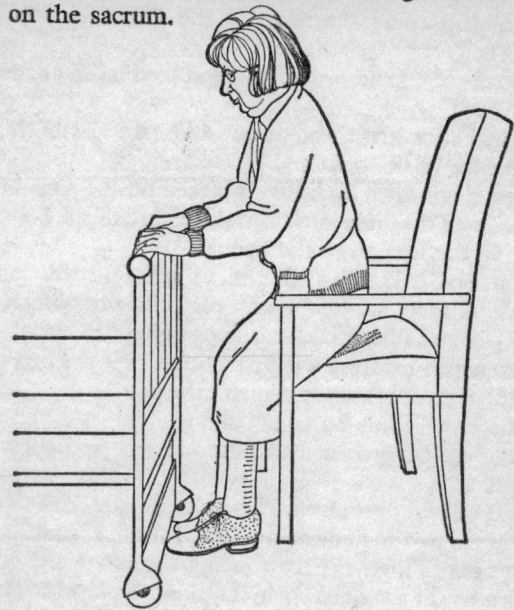

FIG. 4 End of bed exercises

(d) Walking. When the patient begins to walk the best support can be given by two nurses standing one on either side, their inside arms encircling the back of her waist while the patient's hands press down into their outside hands. She should be encouraged to look ahead, not down at her feet, and to take normal steps. When assisting a hemiplegic patient the nurse standing on the affected side can use her own leg to brace the knee when that side takes the weight and as the patient steps forward the nurse can use her own foot to lift the affected foot forward.

Walking with a Zimmer frame. Gradually the patient can learn to hold and lift a walking frame while still being supported by a nurse on either side or by one nurse from behind. Some patients dislike using a walking frame, probably because they

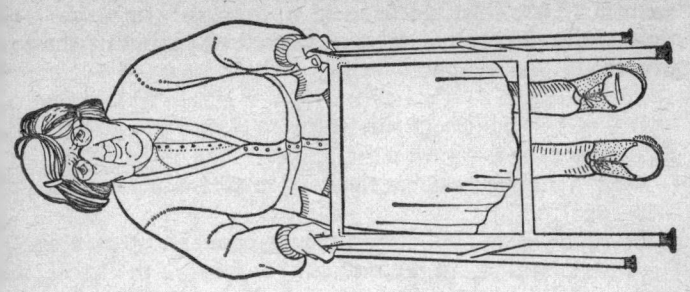

Fig. 5 How to support a patient when she first begins to walk

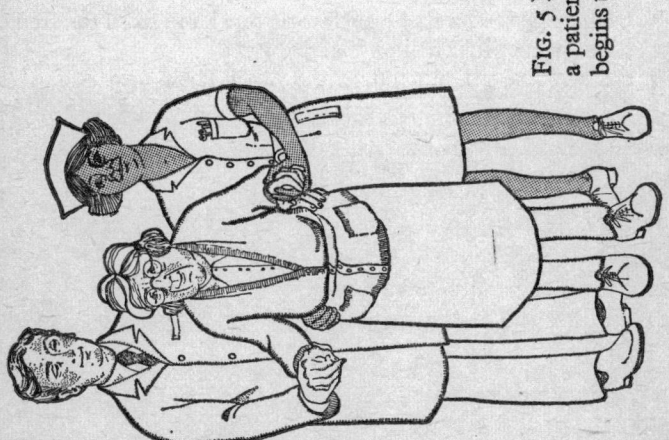

Fig. 6 Walking with a zimmer frame

are using it incorrectly. It is important that they be taught the right way from the beginning. The patient should be shown how to:

1. lift the frame forward and place it a comfortable distance (12–18") ahead (a common fault is to place it too far ahead);
2. step into the frame with the leading foot (the one naturally used to initiate a step, or the unaffected foot in a hemiplegic patient); and
3. bring the other foot forward the distance of a 'step' in front of the first foot but not too near the front of the frame, so that the body is comfortably balanced before starting another step.

Some patients try to hurry these actions by lifting the frame as they are making the step so that it does not give support when it is most needed.

(e) **Sitting down in a chair.** A patient who is still unsteady on her feet and using a walking frame should be shown the simplest way to sit down without the risk of falling, being trained to:

1. walk up to the chair and walk round in a large semi-circle until the chair is behind her;
2. back towards the chair until she can feel the seat with the back of her legs;
3. balance herself before transferring one hand from the frame to the arm of the chair on that side; and
4. transfer the other hand to the other chair arm and with both hands supporting the body lift herself back into the chair.

Although the directions may seem obvious, many elderly people will try to sit while still holding the frame and will fall heavily back into the chair. Others may naturally approach the chair forwards and cannot cope with pushing the frame to one side and turning through a half-circle which will involve transferring the supporting hand from one arm of the chair to the other.

(f) **Getting up from a chair.** The most common error made by the patient is to pull herself up, using the walking frame rather than the arms of the chair. She should:

1. lift herself forward to the edge of the chair seat with her hands on the arms and place her feet firmly on the floor,

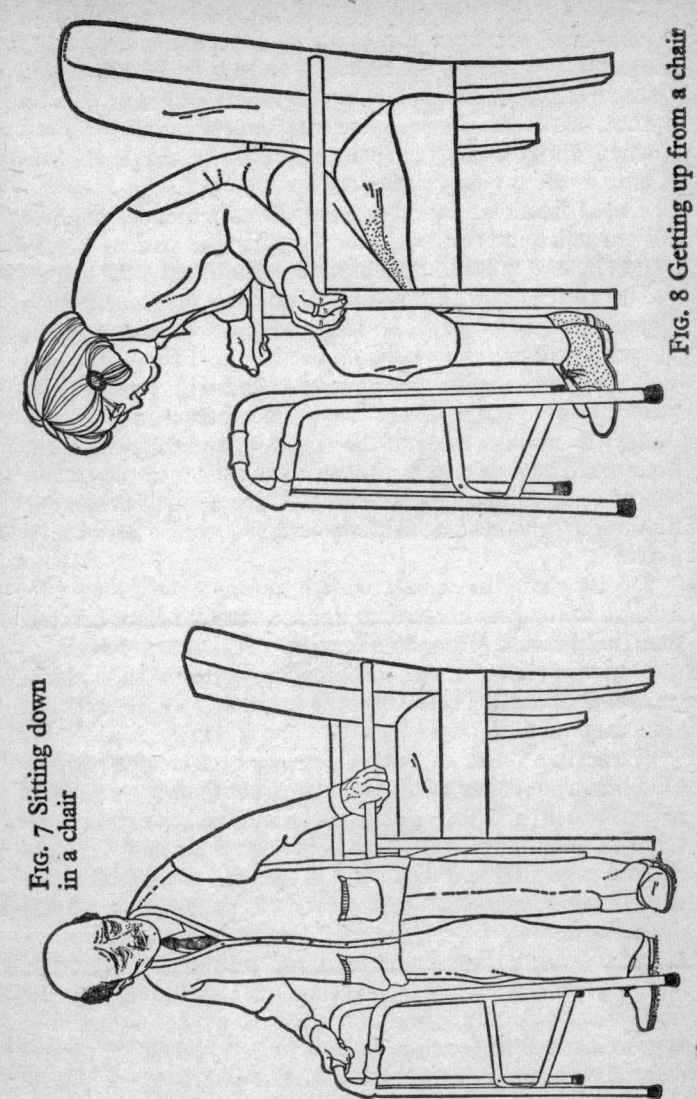

FIG. 7 Sitting down in a chair

FIG. 8 Getting up from a chair

immediately in front of the chair and slightly apart;
2. use the muscles of her buttocks and thighs to lift herself into a standing position, using her hands and arms to press down on the chair arms to give extra impetus; and
3. when upright and well balanced, transfer one hand at a time to the walking frame.

The co-ordination needed for the single movement of standing upright will require practice and at first the patient can be helped by one or two nurses lifting her from under the axillae.

The patient will find getting in and out of a chair more difficult if it is too low. To judge whether a chair is of the correct height the patient should be able to sit right back in it with the lumbar spine well supported and with a right angle formed at both hip and knee joints. The chair should be deep enough to support most of the length of the thighs and the feet should be able to reach the floor. A patient in the correct size of chair will become independent more quickly than one who has to rely on someone for assistance because her chair is too low.

Special chairs are made with a sprung seat which tilts forward as the patient starts to rise and gives an extra boost to the crucial action of standing upright. For a patient whose leg muscles are wasted or whose joints are arthritic such chairs can make all the difference between remaining chairbound and regaining mobility.

(g) Dressing. Once any acute illness has been treated patients can remain out of bed for the greater part of the day, preferably in a day room and they should be encouraged to dress themselves in their day clothes. Getting dressed is not easy for those patients who find it difficult to balance and whose joints are stiff. They will find it easier to put on their clothes sitting down. A woman patient, for example, can put on her underclothes, dress or blouse and skirt and pull on her stockings and knickers while she sits, and then can stand to pull up her knickers and stockings and afterwards to smoothe down her skirt and adjust her clothes. She may need the help of a nurse to support her at first but as her balance improves she will be able to hold on to the bed or a chair with one hand and adjust her clothes with the other. A hemiplegic patient should be shown how to dress by putting the weak limb first into the sleeve or leg of the garment.

For women, a dress that buttons down the front is the easiest to put on, but a skirt with a blouse or cardigan is more versatile. It is important that the patient should feel properly dressed by being encouraged to wear her underclothes. Laundry may be a problem for patients who are infrequently visited, and the hospital volunteer service may be able to help.

Shoes are very important. Ideally all patients should have a pair of laced walking shoes which must be worn when they begin any walking exercises. Slippers may be easier to put on but they do not support the foot and may cause the patient to trip. Some elderly people have feet that are grossly deformed by bunions and callouses and can never get comfortable shoes. Special shoes can be made and fitted by the surgical appliance officer of the hospital service. Other patients, after treatment by the chiropodist, may find their shoes more comfortable.

Aids to dressing. For the patient who lacks the finer movements of the hand through paralysis or arthritis, or whose movements are otherwise limited, there are various ways to make dressing easier. Buttons and hooks can be replaced by Velcro or press studs, openings can be enlarged and skirts cut so that they wrap over. A special aid can make the job of pulling on stockings much easier and an elongated shoe horn and elastic shoe laces can help the patient who cannot bend easily to put on shoes. The Disabled Living Foundation (346 Kensington High Street, London W14) will advise on the different adaptations that can be made to clothes and will know suppliers of clothes suitable for disabled people. The occupational therapist can also help the patient to cope with difficulties in dressing and suggest individual aids.

The role of the physiotherapist

The physiotherapist will plan and undertake the more formal exercises in the rehabilitation programme and every nurse should be familiar with the exercises and equipment used by the physiotherapist so that she will understand the range of activities in which the patient will be involved. Some wards will arrange for each nurse to spend time with the physiotherapist during her ward activities and in the gymnasium, but if this is not regular policy the nurse should ask if it can be arranged. It is important to learn from the physiotherapist the correct way to lift and assist a patient (see also Chapter 7), for the patient may be hurt and the nurse injured if lifting is performed incorrectly.

A programme of exercises conducted by the physiotherapist may involve

passive exercises (already discussed at the beginning of this chapter);

assisted exercises: the patient exercises various muscles with the aid of the physiotherapist who supports the limb or helps to put the muscles through a fuller range of movement; alternatively, the weight of the limb may be supported in a sling suspended above the patient;

exercises against resistance; the patient exercises and strengthens the muscles against a variable resistance, either provided by the physiotherapist herself or by apparatus which uses the mechanical resistance of springs, weights and pulleys; and

balance exercises: balance is extremely important in the rehabilitation of elderly people, some of whom may have developed bad habits of posture and gait and so distort their own balance; factors contributing to poor balance are obesity, osteo-arthritis, Parkinson's Disease, kyphosis, poor eyesight and conditions such as Ménière's Disease which affect the balance mechanism of the inner ear. Lack of confidence may make an elderly person lean forward when walking, taking little hurried steps so that her balance is upset. Relearning to balance is important following a stroke, when a patient not only loses voluntary movement of one side of the body, but may also lose sensation and awareness of the existence of the limbs on the affected side (anosognosia).

Balance exercises, including assisted and resisted exercises, are likely to take place with the patient lying or sitting on a purpose-built plinth covered by a mat and set at a comfortable height for the physiotherapost. These mat exercises give patients increased confidence; because they do not have to concentrate on standing, are less likely to slip and have more space in which to move or roll without falling, they are able to concentrate harder on exercising their muscles. Bad posture and gait may be improved if patients are helped to see their own faults in a mirror and to correct them while they are sitting or walking.

Functional exercises. As muscle strength and co-ordination improve so patients will graduate to more functional exercises. Walking practice may start with walking between parallel bars and from there graduating to a walking (Zimmer) frame, tripod or elbow crutches. Later they may manage with a stick only and finally walk unaided, though they may want to retain the stick for extra confidence. Many patients will return home with a walking frame and it is becoming a more common sight to see elderly people using one when out shopping. The tripod and quadripod are designed for hemiplegic patients unable to grip both sides of a walking frame, who may also be supplied with a below-knee caliper to support the weakened ankle of the affected foot. The aids supplied must be of the right height for the patient; it cannot be expected that a Zimmer frame suitable for a small woman will be comfortable for a tall man. Aids supplied by the physiotherapy department should be clearly labelled with the patient's name so that they are not used by the wrong patient.

Functional exercises will also include getting into and out of bed, sitting down and getting up from a chair, climbing stairs and negotiating doorways with a walking frame. A wheelchair may be provided for the patient unable to walk, as the result of, perhaps, a stroke, arthritis or a serious fracture, and she must be shown how to use it.

Other aids. The physiotherapist will supply the splints needed to support the grossly deformed joints of patients with rheumatoid arthritis and to prevent and correct contractures. These splints are made individually of plaster of paris or of moulded plastic and are bound n place with crepe bandages. The nurse should understand the correct use of such splints as she will be required to fit them at night or for limited periods during the day. Care should be taken that the splints do not cause pressure sores. A patient with a paralysed arm may support it in a sling to prevent undue strain on the ligament of the shoulder joint, and the nurse should make sure that the sling is comfortably adjusted.

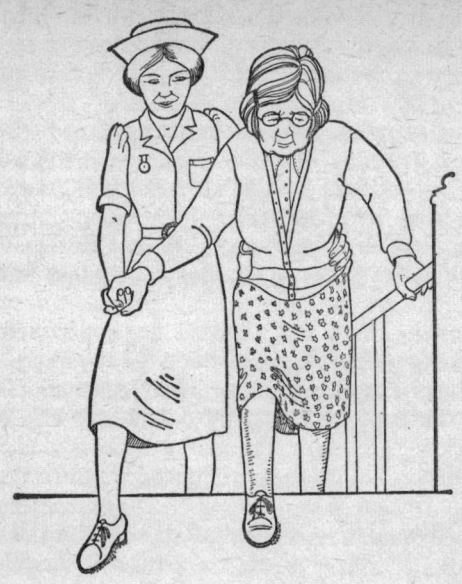

FIG. 9 Practising climbing stairs

Other treatment. Another aspect of the physiotherapist's work is the treatment of deep and necrosed pressure sores with ultra-violet light, usually two or three times each week. The ultra-violet light will hasten the breakdown of slough and clean the infected areas, and the treatment is used in conjunction with appropriate dressings. On treatment days the nurse should work with the physiotherapist so that the dressing can be renewed as soon as the treatment has been given. Local radiant heat from a lamp may also be used to improve the circulation to a superficial sore.

Heat lamps may also be used to treat painful arthritic joints and the nurse may be asked to give this treatment. It is essential that she should understand the length and extent of the treatment and the dangers of overexposure. The ward may be a temporary home for the equipment for such specialised treatment and apparatus must be stored carefully where it cannot be damaged.

The rôle of the occupational therapist

The occupational therapist plays an important part in the rehabilitation of elderly people. Her particular functions in the rehabilitation programme are:

1. To assess the ability of patients to manage the activities of daily living necessary to become independent, and to decide well before discharge whether any special adaptations will be needed in the home. Before discharge, the occupational therapist may visit the patient's home to assess what is needed, and a further visit with the patient may be required to ensure that there are no unforeseen difficulties such as a wheelchair being too wide to go through the doorways. Sometimes these home visits are done by the occupational therapist employed by the local Social Services Department and she will be responsible for getting any adaptations done. In owner-occupied property, adaptations such as fitting a ramp or rails or even an electric hoist should not be a great problem, especially if the patient or her family can help towards the cost. In privately rented or council property there may be legal problems which delay the start of adaptations as well as the difficulty of finding carpenters or builders to do the major works. It is essential to persevere, because in financial terms alone the cost of alterations, however extensive, is likely to be a fraction of the cost of keeping a patient in hospital, and so long as the patient wants to go home and the right equipment and help are made available, the benefits of being independent in one's own home are immeasurable.

2(a). To retrain the patient to simple but important tasks such as dressing, washing and cooking simple meals, and (b) to supply any aids that may make these tasks easier for the patient and to train her in their use.

For example: 'Mrs R., aged 70, lives with her husband and is admitted to hospital with an acute epsiode of long-standing rheumatoid arthritis. After the acute attack has subsided, the joints of her hands and fingers are still extremely painful, and she has difficulty in gripping. She is assessed in the occupational therapy department and supplied with a set of cutlery with handles encased in rubber padding to make them easier to hold. The water taps in her home are to be fitted with levers which can be pushed with the elbows, and her gas taps are similarly adapted. She is shown that a sponge is easier to grip than a flannel and that soap, held in a magnetic holder to the side of the bath is more manageable when washing. As she also has difficulty in lifting her arms to comb her hair, she is supplied with a long handled comb.'

Many of these simple aids and other adaptations to the home can be made by a relative or friend and do not require expensive equipment. Once the principle of the aid is understood it can be tailored to the individual needs of the patient. Aids to dressing have been discussed under 'The Rôle of the Nurse'. Ideally the occupational therapy department should have a simulated bedroom large enough for the furniture to be moved around to represent the patient's own room, and equipped with a domestic bed which is usually lower and narrower than a hospital one. A bathroom and lavatory will be useful to teach the patient the technique of getting in and out of the bath and to try out any aids such as a bath seat or a raised lavatory seat.

Similarly, a kitchen with gas and electric cookers, a sink, and cupboards with shelving of various heights, can be used to assess and teach the patient and to demonstrate the many aids that can be used in the kitchen. There may also be a sitting room for diversional activities.

3. To provide diversional occupation for patients to stimulate their interest and encourage the use of their joints and muscles, especially in the finer movements of the hands. Diversional occupation may be undertaken in groups or individually.

Many elderly people, particularly those living alone, lose interest in most things other than passive entertainment such as watching television or reading the newspaper. In hospital the burden of coping with the day-to-day problems of living is taken from them and this can be a good time to re-interest them in other activities. Apart from the obvious, such as knitting, basket work and various forms of weaving, occupational therapists will be able to encourage patients to paint, cook, do light industrial work or pack items for the hospital's sterile supply department. If these activities are conducted in small groups, conversation is easier between patients working on the same task. Group activities such as bingo sessions, singing and acting allow people to participate in some way despite their disabilities. If these activities are run in conjunction with a day hospital where patients discharged from the ward can attend, or if similar facilities are available in the local authority day centres, the change from hospital to home will be easier for the patient to accept.

Music therapy is a recently developed technique to encourage elderly people to join in group activities. Not only can appropriate music be played to provide the rhythm in group exercise sessions but music can also be used to stimulate imaginative mimes by patients who may be inhibited by formal speech. Old music-hall tunes will stir the memories of older people and encourage them to join in with dancing and singing. Some patients suffering from dysphasia following a stroke have been found to be able to sing clearly when they cannot speak.

The rôle of the speech therapist

Speech therapists are specifically involved in the rehabilitation of patients who have lost some of their ability to comprehend or to communicate (dysphasia) following a stroke (see Chapter 4). Re-training such a patient is a very long task which will involve teaching the patient to use the very simplest words, illustrating them by actions or objects. Relatives can be shown how they can help patients once they have returned home. Unfortunately, many elderly patients suffer from other mental changes following a stroke and they have not always retained their concentration sufficiently to withstand intensive speech therapy. There are rarely sufficient speech therapists to help every patient whose speech has been affected, and younger patients or those less severely affected who are likely to benefit most from the training will be given priority.

Speech therapists may also treat patients with dysarthria,

a mechanical difficulty in speaking that follows a stroke, the onset of Parkinson's disease or multiple sclerosis.

Others involved in the rehabilitation of the patient

Relatives. The relatives have an important part to play in rehabilitation, and their interest in the patient's progress will encourage her to persevere with difficult exercises. Conversely, relatives who do not want the old person to return home may discourage her, perhaps unwittingly, from trying to help herself.

The physiotherapist or occupational therapist may invite a close relative to see what exercises and activities the patient is undertaking in order to understand how the patient is being helped and can continue the exercises upon returning home. Not only must the patient who is discharged from hospital with a walking aid or other appliance be instructed carefully in how to use it but the relative should also be shown so that she can make sure that the aid is being used correctly.

The relatives of patients who have suffered a stroke have an essential part to play in their rehabilitation. Some patients may be able to go home from hospital a few weeks after having had the stroke but in many cases their recovery from its effects will take many months and the relatives must be involved. They can be shown how to exercise paralysed limbs, how to communicate with the patient and help to restore her speech, and how to lift and help her to move. This will involve the relative in attending several sessions with the patient in the physiotherapy or occupational therapy departments before discharge and returning with her to the hospital from time to time to discuss the patient's progress and to learn new exercises.

The social worker is responsible for advising the patient about her social problems and she will be involved in any discussions about the patient's progress and discharge. She may want to interview the patient's relatives and advise them on the help for which they or the patient may be eligible, such as the Constant Attendance Allowance or help towards the cost of adaptations in the home. She will also arrange for the patient to be provided with a home help, meals-on-wheels or other services (see Chapter 9). It is she who will arrange for a patient to be admitted to a local authority or private old people's home, or for the payment of rent due on the patient's house or flat to preserve the tenancy. She has the very difficult task of preserving the patient's link with the community while in hospital.

The chiropodist. Chiropody treatment can make the difference between a patient being chairbound, with all its attendant problems, and being able to walk. Elderly people have great difficulty in attending to their feet, and ingrowing toenails, corns and callouses can be so painful that some will give up walking. Ideally, all patients should be seen by a chiropodist while in hospital, but diabetic patients and those with circulatory disturbances, who are at particular risk of developing gangrene of their toes and feet, should never be treated by an unskilled person with unsuitable tools, and so should be given priority to see the chiropodist.

The hospital chaplain can be an enormous help and comfort to old people in hospital. Unlike the doctors and nurses who must always seem so busy, he has time to sit and talk to patients who may find it easier to discuss their anxieties with him because he is not involved in their everyday care. Any patients who are interested should be encouraged to attend the services in the hospital chapel for, apart from the spiritual benefits of the service, the interest of another activity outside the ward will help towards their return to independence.

Voluntary helpers. Many hospitals have Voluntary Help Schemes and lay people working in the wards provide another link between patients and the outside world. A patient who has no relatives can be 'visited' by one particular volunteer, who can not only be a practical help by shopping and writing letters, but can take a special interest in that patient and her progress. Volunteers may also help with the group activities and provide entertainments in the ward. Anything that will enliven the interest of patients will help towards their rehabilitation.

For Further Reading

Eaton Griffiths, V. *A Stroke in the Family*. Penguin Books, 1970

Hawker, M. *Geriatrics for Physiotherapists and Allied Professions.* Faber, 1974

Ritchie, D. *Stroke!* Faber, 1960

Todd, J. Physiotherapy in the early stages of hemiplegia. (Part 1; The adult hemiplegic). *Physiotherapy*, 1974

Wareham, T. *Return to Independence.* Chest and Heart Association, 1976

9. Return to the Community

The aim of geriatric care, stressed throughout this book, is to enable the patient to return to the community to live as independently as possible. However, the nurse who has previously worked in general medical and surgical wards and who is accustomed to see patients come from their homes and return to them as a matter of course will soon realise that the situation is not so straightforward for the patient discharged from a geriatric ward. The problems facing the elderly patient leaving hospital are partly those faced by any elderly person living in a society which has, over the last 50 years, become much more mobile and is generally less able (which is not to say less willing) to care for its elderly infirm, and partly those arising from the die-hard attitude that lingers among some people that all geriatric patients are 'hopeless cases' requiring long term, custodial care.

An ideal society is able to provide the right accommodation for its elderly members whose own homes become unsuitable; a ground-floor flat, a place in sheltered housing or in a home for the mentally frail would be available when needed. However, with the limited resources available for the care of the elderly such an ideal state does not exist and all too often a patient is discharged from hospital to a home which is unsatisfactory. The alternative course is to compel the patient to remain in hospital, which is contrary to the aims of treatment and mobilisation and naturally prevents other elderly people from being admitted. It would also be an environment more unsuitable for the patient in the long term than the one to which she is returning.

The problem is not one for the doctor, social worker or ward sister alone. Every nurse working for the rehabilitation of elderly people will find herself confronted with the dilemma of seeing a patient discharged to a home which is highly unsuitable, often against the wishes of the patient's relatives and even of the patient. A nurse new to the geriatric ward can become distressed and confused by the strength of feeling generated by the issues involved in discharging a patient. She may take the brunt of the relatives' anger on finding their elderly mother or aunt is due to be discharged. She cannot 'take sides' in the issue. She must recognise the rights of the patient and the problems of the relatives. She must understand the limitations of the solutions available and above all she must not jeopardise the patient's planned discharge by an ill-chosen remark to a relative such as 'of course they won't expect your mother to come home, she could never manage' which the relative may accept as the doctor's decision.

This is not to suggest that all relatives are unwilling for their mothers, aunts or other elderly relatives to be discharged. Many devoted daughters, sons, nieces and even more distant relatives, as well as the husband or wife of the patient, go to enormous lengths to help and support an old person, but some elderly people can be extremely trying and at their worst can totally disrupt a family by their need for constant attention or by their selfish demands. It is understandable that if an old person has been ill for some time before admission to hospital and the strain of caring for her has become severe enough to threaten the health of the family, the relatives will see in the hospital a solution to their problem – a place where 'Mum can be put away' to relieve them of their burden. Their previous experience of caring for the old person may make them unwilling to accept the responsibility again.

In contrast, many elderly people given suitable support, are quite capable of living in the community but neighbours, friends and relatives may think otherwise and try to insist that the patient should not be allowed home. Their reasons may be telling: 'She's always turning the gas on and forgetting to light it, she'll blow us all up one day'; 'She'll have a fall one day and no one will know about it'; 'She's filthy, the house is full of mice'. Keeping a neighbourly eye on elderly people can be a time consuming tie, particularly if they do not appreciate the efforts made on their behalf.

In any decision about their future, one thing is paramount:

the right of patients to choose for themselves where they shall live within the limitations of the choice available. For those patients who feel able to return to their own homes, every effort should be made to allow them to do so. A landlord, for instance, has no right to evict an elderly person while in hospital, provided the rent is paid, however unfit or unable to return he thinks that person may be.

The only situation to which a patient may be unable to return is to the home of a relative. Sons and daughters no longer have a legal obligation to house or care for their parents. In the rare case where the relatives literally lock the door against them, they are acting within the law, whatever the patients' wishes may be.

Ideally, the patient and interested relatives should discuss the whole question of discharge with the doctor, social worker, ward sister and perhaps a health visitor from the community, so that everyone is aware of the problems that may arise and how they may be overcome and also recognises the real limitation of the choice of accommodation available. Much misunderstanding and recrimination would be avoided if relatives could participate in all discussions on the patient's future from the time of admission to the ward.

Planned discharge

An elderly person's discharge from hospital must be carefully planned, bearing in mind the sort of problems that have been outlined above. The social worker may have prepared a social report about the patient, describing her home and its drawbacks, the help received and the degree of contact with relatives and friends. This will be the basis for discussion; questions can then be posed as to the patient's needs:

1. Can the patient continue to live in the same place as before admission to hospital?

If the answer is 'yes':

(*a*) What help can be expected from relatives and neighbours and what domiciliary services will be needed?

(*b*) Will some form of day care help the patient to live independently? Will it be needed for a limited time or indefinitely? How frequently will it be needed?

2. If the old home is unsuitable:
   (*a*) Will the support of warden-supervised accommodation be needed?
   (*b*) Will the fuller support of an old people's home be needed? What sort of home would be appropriate?
   (*c*) Has the patient relatives who are willing to look after her?

The majority of patients will return to their own accommodation, however unsuitable, because as will be seen, an alternative is so difficult to find. Many elderly people will be able to cope better in the home they know and where they have roots in the community; moving to more 'ideal' accommodation may be an intolerable change.

In order to help answer these questions, the doctor will need to know from the occupational therapist how well the patient can manage the activities of daily living and from the physiotherapist and nursing staff her progress in any rehabilitation programme. When it is impossible for the patient to return home it may take several months to find suitable alternative accommodation, and even years if the only suitable place is in a local authority old people's home. In some cases temporary accommodation may be found in a relative's home. It is therefore important that a patient's discharge should be discussed well before she is fully fit to leave hospital, and once a provisional date has been fixed for discharge the relatives must be told immediately. The ward sister should discuss with the nursing staff the social situation and discharge plans for all patients so that they are informed sufficiently to be able to talk to the patients about their future and encourage them to become more independent.

Extended discharge

For patients who have been in hospital for a long time and have come to depend upon the hospital for food and daily care (no matter how physically capable they may be) the shock of the transition to living in the community may be very great. It is possible to extend their period of discharge in various ways so that it is a gradual process and they are able to acclimatise themselves to the changed way of life.

1. *Experimental day or weekend at home*
Patients may be allowed home for the day accompanied by an occupational therapist to see how well they can manage (see Chapter 8, Rehabilitation) or for an experimental weekend, in which case the home nurse may be asked to visit to see how they are coping.

Experimental time at home will reveal any difficulties that may prevent the patient living at home until some alterations are made, such as to a door that will not open widely enough to allow a walking frame to pass through. It will also give the patient confidence in her ability to manage, knowing that at the end of the experimental period she can return to the hospital and will not suddenly be left on her own to cope as best she can. These experimental periods can be repeated several times before the patient is finally discharged.

It may be necessary, after their trial period at home, to allow patients more time in hospital to improve their mobility before they return home permanently. In the rare case where a patient shows that she cannot manage, alternative accommodation can be found without precipitating another crisis which will bring the patient back to hospital for a further lengthy period of rehabilitation.

2. *The halfway house*
Some geriatric departments have, as part of their progressive care facilities (see Chapter 5: The Geriatric Department), a unit where patients learn to live more independently, while still under the supervision of the nursing staff and from where they can be discharged home when they are sufficiently able. A halfway house differs from the conventional convalescent home in that it may be in or near the hospital, so patients may continue to attend the physiotherapy and occupational therapy department and the day hospital. The time spent in the halfway house will vary from a few days to several weeks according to the patients' needs. In many respects the halfway house is similar to the old people's home where the residents are expected to get up, dress themselves, eat together and perhaps join together in communal activities and housework.

The halfway house may allow the patients an opportunity

to cater for themselves, including cooking, budgeting and even shopping. This can be an invaluable experience for people who are anxious to return home but lack confidence because of the length of their stay in hospital. From this supervised independence it is a short step to their own home, particularly if they are able to have a telephone or an alarm system installed.

3. *The day hospital*
The role of the day hospital is discussed fully in Chapter 5 (The Geriatric Department). Some of the patients attending will have been newly discharged from hospital, and others may be helped to settle back into their own homes if they know that they can attend the day hospital daily or once or twice a week and there find the companionship and help they have been used to in hospital. Their progress towards independence can be assessed and they can continue to attend the physiotherapy and occupational therapy departments. Once the support of the hospital is no longer thought necessary, attendance at a local authority day centre may be arranged (see below).

Domiciliary services
Once the patients' discharge has been arranged a decision must be reached about services they will need to help them to live independently. Whether patients return to their own homes, a relative's home, to sheltered housing or a community old people's home they may still need some outside help. These services must be arranged before the patients leave hospital so that the support is forthcoming during the crucial first few days at home. The social worker or ward sister generally arrange these services with the local authority or with the community nursing services.

Services provided by the area health authority
The primary medical care of any patient is provided by the general practitioner, usually working in a group practice from a surgery or health centre. In the majority of cases he will be able to treat his patients without having to refer them to a hospital specialist. He is responsible for the day-to-day health of his

patients, and many of those visiting him or requesting home visits will be elderly. To make his work more effective, a team has been built up around him, usually consisting of the health visitor, the home nurse, the midwife, auxiliary nursing staff, and in some cases a privately employed practice nurse and a social worker. The members of this Primary Care Team will work together, discuss individual cases and refer patients to the appropriate member of the team as necessary. The doctor, health visitor and home nurse will all visit elderly people and if their knowledge of these patients is pooled, the preventive aspect of geriatric care in the community will be greatly enhanced.

General practitioner. When patients are discharged, a letter giving a summary of their illness and treatment while in hospital and particulars of their present treatment, including any arrangements for out-patient appointments, will be sent to their general practitioners, followed by a more detailed report. Most general practitioners like to visit their patients soon after their discharge from hospital and, depending on each patient's need, will continue to visit regularly or arrange for the health visitor attached to the practice to do so. After he has assessed how they are managing at home, he may recommend further domciliary help and vary their medications.

General practitioners will differ in the amount of time they allocate to the routine visiting of their elderly patients. Some try to visit every three months, others may arrange a yearly examination, or may only see the elderly when requested, as with any other patient.

Home nurse. The home nurse (district nurse), a large proportion of whose patients are elderly, provides a nursing service in the home. She will do any dressings needed, such as for colostomies and varicose ulcers; give injections, for example of insulin or Vitamin B_{12}; wash patients or help them to get in and out of bed and settle them for the day or night. The frequency of her visits will depend on the patients' needs; it may vary from a once weekly bath to visiting three times a day to give medications.

Above all, because the home nurse visits her patients regularly she is in a position to make a continuous assessment of their progress and report any deterioration in their condition to the general practitioner. As she has a definite task to do for each patient she is usually made very welcome and quickly becomes a friend of all the family. She can often advise on diet, aids, and the services or organizations that can make the patient's (and her relatives') life more comfortable.

As more people are being cared for in the community, greater demands are being made on the home nurse, so that some of the more straightforward tasks such as bathing an elderly person are carried out by nursing auxiliaries.

Nursing aids. A home nurse will arrange with the local authority or the area health authority to supply any special aids that the patient may need, such as a hoist, a backrest, bed blocks or a commode, unless the occupational therapist has already done this before the patient left hospital. The British Red Cross Society also has centres from which equipment can be supplied on loan. The home nurse will also arrange, if necessary, for a regular supply of incontinence pads to be delivered to the patient.

Night sitter service. Some area health authorities run a night sitter service, using nurses, nursing auxiliaries or volunteers as the situation requires. It must, of necessity, be a very short-term service, because the cost of providing one nurse for a patient is high, but it is particularly useful where a person is too ill to be moved to hospital, or is terminally ill and does not wish to leave home. A night sitter may provide holiday relief for a relative or support a family where the elderly person is particularly confused. The scope of this type of service is at present very limited, but it is a scheme which, if greatly expanded, could allow many more elderly people to remain in the community.

Health visitor. The health visitor, who is a state-registered nurse with some midwifery experience and a year's education and training in the social aspects of nursing and preventive medicine, may visit the elderly person in hospital and again when she has returned home, especially where no home nurse is visiting. She is skilled in assessment and she will ensure that her client is able to manage and has all the help needed, and will advise on diet, minor health problems and any general difficulties with pensions and benefits. The health visitor is normally attached to a group practice and, like the home nurse, can report any changes in the old person's condition to the general practitioner. Some health visitors specialise in visiting the elderly and may be attached to a geriatric department. They, particularly, will be able to see the patient both in hospital and again at home, and may also visit relatives to discuss with them any problems that they may have about the old person's care. These geriatric liaison health visitors will have specialised knowledge of the community care of the elderly, particularly from the medical point of view, and will be able to give advice on the specific problems of old people to their colleagues who visit all age groups.

Services provided by the local authority (County, Borough and District Councils)
Home help. The home help, with the home nurse, is the backbone of the domiciliary services for the elderly. The home help service is run by the local authority as part of the Social Services Department and, because it is paid for with money raised by the rates, its extent varies greatly from authority to authority. Home helps work mainly for old people, and will do housework, shopping, collect the pension and perhaps prepare a meal or make the old person a cup of tea. Many do far more for their elderly clients than is required of them and some will return in their own time in the evenings or at weekends when they know the old person will have no other help. As her visits tend to be lengthy (an hour or more), the home help is company for the old person. She will also be able to see how well her client manages and if there is any deterioration in her ability to cope, she can report back to her supervisor, who in turn can notify the general practitioner or social worker.

A home help may visit as often as twice a day or as infrequently as once a fortnight according to the old person's needs, which are assessed by a supervisor. Payment varies from authority to authority, but old people receiving supplementary pension usually pay nothing; others pay according to their means, up to the full cost of the home help. The service may be provided for a limited time until the patient can manage, or it may continue indefinitely.

Meals-on-wheels. The Meals-on-Wheels service is also paid for by the local authority but in many areas the service is run by the W R V S, whose volunteers drive the vans and deliver the meals or serve at the luncheon clubs for the elderly. Meals-on-wheels are delivered almost exclusively to the elderly housebound and the cost and extent of the service varies from area to area. Some areas are able to provide – for a limited number of people – a meal every day, while in other areas meals may be delivered only twice a week. The cost to the old person varies from about 5p to 20p, but in some areas it is free. The meals may be cooked in a central kitchen and served on plates from a delivery van but more and more use is being made of pre-cooked meals in foil containers which only need heating.

The meals-on-wheels service ensures that elderly people get a regular hot meal (which in many cases provides most of the essential nutrients in the diet) at low cost, and that someone visits them regularly. One of the regrets of many of the deliverers of the meals is that they cannot spend longer with the old people but they do at least see them regularly and can report if they need help. If an old person does not open the door as usual, the social worker or the police will be told and, if necessary, the house is broken into.

The meal service also provides meals at luncheon clubs for the elderly, which are held in community centres and church halls. These clubs not only provide cheap meals but are places where old people can meet, and will often form the basis of a social club with other activities, such as coach trips and talks. As any elderly people can attend the luncheon club, it can become an event around which they can plan their day and for which they must make an effort to get out. If a regular attender at the club fails to come for a few days, one of the organisers will arrange for that person to be visited.

Social workers. Social workers are either hospital or community-based. The hospital social worker may visit at home or refer the patient to her community-based colleague. Social workers visit people with essentially social problems, such as those involving relatives and relationships within the family, legal pro lems of tenancies, and money and housing problems. They will also give advice on the services which are available and assess the suitability (with the help of medical reports) of a person applying for admission to a local authority old people's home or sheltered housing, whether directly from hospital or from home.

A social worker may help elderly people to apply for a supplementary pension, or benefits such as a heating grant, but she should not be confused with officers of the Department of Health and Social Security who may also visit elderly people to discuss their application for benefit and assess their means.

Community occupational therapist. Some local authorities employ occupational therapists to visit elderly people at home and advise on aids and alterations that could help to make their homes easier to run. Their work is discussed in the previous chapter (Rehabilitation).

There is, of course, considerable overlap between the work of the social worker, the health visitor and the community occupational therapist. The social worker has the greater statutory powers, the health visitor has expert medical knowledge and the occupational therapist the skills needed to equip the elderly with suitable aids. Until there is one body of people with statutory obligation to visit all elderly people and to co-ordinate the work of the specialist visitors, this overlap is likely to continue.

Laundry service. A laundry service for the incontinent is provided in some areas. The cost varies and the old person is usually required to have a good stock of linen as the laundry is only collected once or twice a week. It is an invaluable service in the situation where a daughter is working and looking after an elderly incontinent mother, or where an elderly person, while quite able to live alone, cannot manage much heavy washing.

Telephone. Some social service departments will arrange for an old person to have a telephone installed, when they feel that no other alarm system would be suitable. The department will usually pay the quarterly rental but the old person pays for the calls.

The local authority may also provide other domiciliary services to make life easier for old people but which are not essential immediately they leave hospital.

Chiropody. Most local authorities provide a subsidised chiropody service for all old age pensioners which helps to keep them mobile and free from corns and sores. The elderly with diabetes and poor peripheral circulation should have priority. The service operates mainly at clinics but the domiciliary chiropodist will, if necessary, make home visits.

Library. Some local authority libraries provide a domiciliary service where a member of the staff or a volunteer will visit an elderly person at home every two or three weeks to change her books. This is an important contact with the outside world for housebound people for whom reading plays a large part in their lives.

Holidays. Social Service Departments and some voluntary organisations arrange low-cost holidays for elderly people, usually in the less busy season at holiday camps or guest houses. Some authorities have their own holiday homes. These holidays are intended for the mobile, but some clubs for the disabled elderly will arrange holidays abroad.

Voluntary help
Old people's welfare committees. Most areas have a committee to co-ordinate the work of local organisations for the elderly and these old people's welfare committees, usually financed by a local government grant, are in turn affiliated to the National Old People's Welfare Council, known as Age Concern. The local committees run voluntary visiting schemes, where individuals help with shopping, writing letters, or gardening on an informal basis. They may also run a Good Neighbour Service (see below). The committees may also be responsible for running clubs, classes and entertainments, as well as fund raising activities. Information about local old

people's welfare committees can be found at the local council offices.

Good neighbour service. This scheme provides untrained people, often housewives, who visit an old person regularly and do some small service, such as collecting her pension, making a cup of tea or helping the person to bed in the evening. For this assistance they are paid a small sum to emphasise that the service is regular and to distinguish them from voluntary visitors.

Other groups. Task Force, Community Service Volunteers, churches, youth groups and schools may all be sources of voluntary help for elderly people. Many secondary schools now include social studies in their final-year curricula and this may involve some visiting of old people by pupils.

Day care
It may be possible for old people to live at home, either in their own home or with a relative, provided that some form of day care can be arranged. The rôle of the day hospital has already been discussed in this respect but it should only care for old people for a limited time – perhaps a few months – and it is intended primarily for those patients who need the facilities of the hospital (physiotherapy, occupational therapy, etc). There are, however, other old people whose daily care needs some supervision, either because their mobility is limited or their tendency to fall or to forget things makes it difficult to leave them alone, who nevertheless wish to live at home and can be cared for in the evenings and at night. A case history illustrates this situation.

'Mrs F. lives with her son, who leaves for work each day at 8 am and returns at 6 pm. Following a stroke, for which she was in hospital for 8 weeks, Mrs F. can walk only with a Tripod aid and she can neither lift things nor prepare food. She has had several falls since coming home but does not like being confined to a chair. She is mentally alert, although her speech has been affected by her stroke. She enjoys company but gets few visitors, and living at the top of a block of flats she has little of interest to watch. Consequently she has recently become depressed and her anxiety has made it all the more difficult for her son to leave her. She attended the day hospital for two months after coming out of hospital and she feels she would be happier if she were able to get away from the flat and be with other people for some days of the week.'

Day centres. Day centres, run by local authorities or charities, provide care for their members throughout the day with meals and communal activities. The day centre is more than a luncheon or social club because the elderly person can spend all day there and as transport is usually provided, people who have previously been housebound can attend. Attendance may be once or twice a week or every day.

Some day centres provide light industrial work and occupational therapy for their members, as well as such activities as drama groups and art sessions. A chiropodist and a hairdresser may visit regularly. Inter-club activities and outings allow a relatively immobile old person to go visiting and meet new people.

Inevitably, there are rarely enough places in day centres to keep pace with the demand. Transport also is often a limiting factor, for, as with the day hospital, the journey to the day centre may be a long one. Some day centres cater specifically for the handicapped, while others allow any elderly person to attend but may reserve some places for people needing transport.

Clubs and classes. Apart from the day centres there are many clubs and organisations for elderly people run by churches or charities, or based at community centres. The social worker will be able to tell patients about them before they leave hospital. Luncheon clubs have already been mentioned and through these an old person may be able to join a social club. Many adult education classes are held during the day. They provide stimulating interest and the opportunity for old people to mix with people outside their own age group.

Clubs cannot offer the same help to a handicapped person as will a day centre but they do provide the interest and opportunity to meet other people that many elderly people need, but may not have explored before going into hospital.

Old people's homes. Some local authority old people's homes accept elderly people on a daytime only basis, giving them the advantage of care and companionship during the day and enabling them to return home at night.

Permanent care in the community

Some patients discharged from hospital will be unable to return to their own homes, because they are either too physically or mentally frail to live alone or their home is quite unsuitable. It may be possible to find alternative accommodation for these patients.

A more suitable home. Where the home of an old person is unsuitable it may be possible to find a more convenient place. A council flat up several flights of stairs may be exchanged for a ground floor flat, or the old family home may be sold and a modern bungalow bought instead. In some cases the local authority will buy a large old house for development and rehouse the owner in an old person's bungalow.

Unfortunately, most of these arrangements take many months to complete and some temporary accommodation may have to be found for the old person in the meanwhile. There is also the danger, as with any elderly people moving house, that she will find it difficult to adapt to a new home, especially if it is a new neighbourhood.

Moving to live with relatives. The relatives of a patient unable to return to her own home may be willing to accept her into their home. Ideally, any decision of this sort should be agreed on by all members of the family (including the children) and fully discussed with the geriatrician and the social worker. What on the face of it seems to be an admirable solution may in the long term lead to friction and great unhappiness. This is especially likely where accommodation is very cramped or where the family has had irregular contact with the old person, perhaps a family visit every few months when everyone has been at their most agreeable. The relatives offering hospitality may themselves be in their 40s or 50s, with adolescent or grown-up children of their own. This should be a time of new-found freedom and prosperity for them, with, perhaps, the wife taking up a job or career again. The added responsibility of an elderly relative will limit this freedom and may cause bitter resentment.

This is not to say that an elderly person can never successfully live with relatives but it is something that must be carefully planned and the family should be given all the support possible, including perhaps the offer of a holiday bed in hospital for the old person for two weeks during the summer, when the wards are likely to be less busy.

A relative may be willing to accept the old person on the understanding that it is only until more permanent accommodation can be found; this may be a difficult undertaking, because the waiting lists for places in sheltered housing or old people's homes are often very long. Any arrangement of this sort is best considered as a long-term one.

Sheltered housing. Sheltered housing, already briefly mentioned in Chapter 3, is particularly suitable for old people who are mentally able but whose mobility is restricted so that they cannot cope in their own houses, but can manage to live in a well-planned small flat, bedsitting room or bungalow. Some of these housing schemes are provided by the local housing authority, either incorporated into new housing estates or built in conjunction with old people's homes, and others by charities or housing associations such as Help the Aged. The rents are reasonable and if the pensioner has only a small income a supplementary pension is usually available to help towards the rent and leave enough to live on.

The advantage of sheltered housing schemes is that an elderly person can live there independently, knowing that help is available, if needed, because each dwelling is connected to an alarm system and the warden visits daily. Domiciliary services are available as for anyone in need in the community (see above) although some housing schemes may provide domestic help. Some schemes will include a communal dining room for residents which perhaps will be used also as a luncheon club for other elderly people. Unfortunately, there are not nearly enough sheltered housing units available to satisfy present demand.

Homes for the elderly. An old people's home was at one time considered to be the answer for any elderly person who could not or did not wish to go on living in her own home (as previously mentioned in Chapter 3). The National Assistance Act (1948) empowered local authorities to provide homes for the elderly and anyone could request a place. Nowadays, places are so limited that an old person may have to wait for several years.

Even the best-run homes tend to be institutionalised, and while the residents can come and go as they please it is usually impossible for them to entertain their friends in private, and they are constantly thrown into the company of people whom they may not like. The common picture of an old people's home is one of the residents all sitting around silently asleep or gazing apathetically out of the window. Even when activities are arranged, many choose not to join in. Curiously, men seem to adapt better to an institutionalised life than women, possibly because they tend to be less physically handicapped and can more easily follow their own pursuits such as walking, visiting the library or pub or watching sport; a woman, however, who has been accustomed to running her own home all her life suddenly finds she is deprived of responsibility. A few people welcome the prospect of community life and will willingly give up their responsibility for cooking, housework and shopping. Homes for the elderly do, however, fulfil a need for those who are physically too frail, or mentally too lacking in confidence to live alone.

Local authority homes vary in size and style. Some of the older ones are situated in what originally were workhouses and may be very large, with dormitory accommodation. Others may be large, converted houses which usually means the residents must be mobile and able to climb stairs. The newer, purpose-built homes provide a bedroom for each resident and the policy is to limit the size of these homes to about thirty residents. Attitudes may vary for several reasons, even in the same area, so that one home will accept residents who are incontinent and need assistance with dressing, while another may only accept completely mobile residents, which is clearly not catering adequately for the groups that need residential care. Some local authorities are building homes for the mentally frail, who in most cases need more supervision than is found in the usual old people's home. Very often the factor that limits the type of resident a home can accept is the availability of staff. Most homes have one or two trained nurses and the matron will be qualified in residential care, but at night only one or two assistants may be on duty.

Local authority old people's homes are the responsibility of the Social Service Department and the application for a place in a home is made through a social worker. A medical report will be necessary, which, if the patient is in hospital, will also include a report from the occupational therapist and the physiotherapist. The cost of a place will depend upon the old person's income but a pensioner receiving the state pension will be given a small allowance for her personal needs. As the waiting period for a place is often very long the patient, or more likely her relatives, may look around for some alternative accommodation.

Charitable residential homes. Various national and local charities and trusts run homes for old people. The conditions for admission vary; some may accept any applicant while for others it may be necessary for the applicant to belong to an organisation or to live in a certain area. Some homes are for one sex only, and others may refuse to allow the resident to bring any of her own possessions. The cost of these homes varies but is usually similar to that of local authority homes. The social worker will know what homes are available locally or a list can be obtained from the Social Services Department.

Private residential homes. These homes, which, like those provided by charities must be registered with the local authority, are variously called nursing homes, guest houses, eventide homes or rest homes. The cost of a place in these homes varies enormously but all are beyond the means of the old person receiving just the state pension, and the facilities are frequently insufficient to provide a reasonable, permanent home for an old person. Some homes have no provision for nursing care, and where the fees are low the diet may be poor and heating minimal.

Unfortunately, some of the cheaper private homes are used by the relatives of elderly people as the only available solution to their own burden of caring for the old person and so they may not inspect the homes thoroughly or care about the facilities offered. One of the very sad aspects of care of the elderly is the number of single people without a family and with only a small pension or annuity, who live in these often inadequate homes, because they have no alternative.

Foster homes. Some local authorities and voluntary societies have recently set up schemes to find foster homes for the elderly in the same way that such homes are found for children. It is obviously important that a family willing to accept an old person should be carefully screened and the old person selected to suit them. The ideal situation might be that of a family where the children have grown up and are away from home, and the house is now too large for the parents who, both still leading active lives, are willing to share some of their home with an old person and provide some care, as they might for an elderly relative. Payment is made by the local authority which accepts responsibility for the old person if the arrangement should break down.

For Further Reading

Francis, G. *Caring for the Elderly*, Heinemann, 1973
Goldberg. *Helping the Aged*. National Institute for Social Work Training, 1970
Norton, D. *Looking after Old People at Home*. N C S S, 1963
Rudinger, E. *Arrangements for Old Age*. Consumers Association, 1970
Stewart, M. *My BrothersKeeper*. Health Horizons, 1968
Townsend, P. *The Last Refuge*. Routledge & Kegan Paul, 1962

10. Geriatric Care – The Present and the Future

The story of the growth of geriatric care in the last 30 years has been remarkable for while developments in other fields of medicine have been towards greater specialisation, more intricate surgery and more potent medicine, geriatric care has diversified, using well established methods of medical treatment and rehabilitation. A philosophy of geriatric care has developed as the needs of elderly patients have come fully to be recognised. The characteristics of this approach have been introduced throughout this book. Firstly came the recognition that many elderly people in long-stay wards suffered from conditions that were treatable; secondly came the realisation that elderly patients needed more than a specific course of medical treatment to make them fit enough to return home to live – they needed rehabilitation. Thirdly, progressive care developed to make full use of the resources available and to provide the right environment for the patient in the course of her treatment and rehabilitation, and fourthly, co-operation between the hospital and the community health and social services has come about as the need grew for supportive services for the elderly patient at home.

Despite these advances in the care of elderly people, there is no cause for complacency. There are still far too many patients in the long-stay wards of geriatric and psychiatric hospitals, whose condition is far from satisfactory. The plight of some of these patients was dramatically highlighted in 1967 with the publication of the report 'Sans Everything – a case to answer'.* As a result of this report and the outcry that followed its publication, the then Minister of Health set up the Hospital Advisory Service to examine the care given in all long-stay hospitals throughout the country. Its members include a

---

*Robb, B. (1967). *Sans Everything – a Case to Answer*. Nelson

doctor, a senior administrative nurse, a clinical nurse and a hospital administrator who visit each hospital and present a confidential report of their findings and recommendations directly to the Secretary of State for Health and Social Security after discussions held at the hospital concerned. The hospital must act upon the recommendations and report their intentions to the Secretary of State. In many cases a lack of resources and finance to improve buildings and recruit staff means that improvement is limited, but where a lack of communication or a poor deployment of staff appears to be the problem, improvements should occur. Many long-stay hospitals have almost insurmountable problems of inadequate, outdated accommodation, insufficient trained staff and a disinterested community offering no support. Only when these difficulties are continually highlighted by the published reports of the Hospital Advisory Service (in which individual hospitals are not identified) will the government and the public realise the overwhelming need for more money to be spent on long-stay care.

In the health care districts where the geriatric services have been developed, the improvement in the quality of care has been dramatic. The status of geriatric care in the medical world will grow as more and more doctors and qualified nurses accept the challenge of caring for the elderly and improving their quality of life. It is unlikely that there will ever be sufficient nurses and para-medical staff to provide a universally high standard of care in all wards and units of geriatric departments, for the proportion of elderly within the community will continue to rise for at least another twenty years, and with greater recognition of the rehabilitative function of geriatric treatment, more elderly patients from other hospital wards (e g orthopaedic and ophthalmic wards) will be transferred to the geriatric department before going home. It is therefore essential that such resources as there are should be used most effectively.

Research and work-study are important if the most effective use is to be made of the limited resources available. Until recent years, nursing practice has often consisted of a somewhat haphazard approach combining traditional methods with common sense. Dwindling finance and the need to raise standards of care means that research must play an important part in highlighting the deficiencies of everyday nursing techniques and showing where improvements can be made. But research is of no value unless its findings are read, understood and widely applied. Every practising nurse should make a point of reading the nursing journals, which carry reports of research findings and the reviews in the journals will tell her of larger research projects, the reports of which may be found in schools of nursing and general libraries. Good nursing research is not dull, dry stuff for academics, it is relevant and applicable to everyday nursing. In a well-functioning geriatric unit, the team of doctors, nurses and para-medical staff should be prepared to discuss and implement the findings of research, whether it be a new method of lifting or a new treatment for pressure sores.

In the future, co-operation between the hospital and community is likely to be more extensive as the primary care team will be playing the major part in the care of old people. Greater emphasis must be put on the prevention of ill health among the elderly in the community and all members of the primary care team can contribute: the doctor by visiting all his elderly patients on some regular basis and by holding routine check-up clinics for the over 60s on the lines of the Child Health Clinics; the health visitor by routine visits to all old people on a system interrelated with the doctor's of, for instance, a yearly, six-monthly or three-monthly visit depending on the patient's age and health; and the home nurse by using her visits to advise and educate while treating her elderly patients. The health visitor will be able to use her skills as an educator by giving talks to old people's clubs and groups and by establishing her own groups in the surgery or health centre for talks and discussions both for the elderly and for relatives caring for old people. The primary care team will be able to draw on the expertise of the geriatrician, physiotherapist, occupational therapist and dietician to extend their range of health education. Health education can be entertaining and amusing if well prepared and supplemented with a variety of aids. Elderly people have time to learn and even if many seem to hold unchangeable attitudes, the majority at least will appreciate the attention paid to them and know to whom to turn when the need arises.

The family doctors are now extending their care into the long stay wards of the community hospitals and pressure on the service will mean more experimentation with different types of care; more day care in day hospitals and centres, more residential homes for the mentally ill and physically handicapped and hospital care for five days a week. Nevertheless, despite these changes the main burden of care is unlikely to shift from the relatives, friends and neighbours of old people and, indeed, as more community projects develop, more people may come to give readily some of their time to help their elderly neighbours. Unless there is a major change in government policy, many elderly people will continue to live on an income that is barely adequate.

By the end of her geriatric experience the nurse in training will have begun to appreciate the developments that have already taken place in this field, and will be aware of the vital need for further expansion, and she will come away with a more positive idea of geriatric care which will be reflected in her approach to all patients, many of whom will be elderly.

Index

ACCIDENTS, IN THE HOME, 63-64
  in the street, 21, 64
  in the ward, 124, 125
  prevention, 64, 65, 124
  reporting, 125
Adaptations in the home, 147
Adult education, 20, 166
Affective disorders, 56-57
Ageing, 4-10, 63
Aids for the incontinent
  patient, 112-113
  in the home, 148
  provided by the home nurse, 160
  to dressing, 143
  to feeding, 120
  to the relief of pressure, 106
  to walking, 145
Alarm systems, 61
Amputation, 37-38
Anaemia, 45-48
  hypoplasia of the bone marrow, 48
  iron deficiency, 45-46
  pernicious, 46-48
Angina pectoris, 33
Anosognosia, 28, 144
Apex beat, 32
Aphasia, 28
Arthritis, osteo-, 41-42
  rheumatoid, 42-44
    nursing care of patient with, 43
Area Health Authority, services provided by, 158-161
Assessment ward, 73-74
Atheroma, 26
Atherosclerosis, 26
Atrial fibrillation, 32, 35, 49
Aural wax, 8

BASAL GANGLIA, 27, 30
Bed, cradle, 43, 106
  getting into, 137
  getting out of, 135, 137
Bereavement, 58, 99
Bladder, 65-69
Blindness, 8, 93-95
Blood pressure, see
  hypertension and hypotension
  transfusion, 48-49
Bone marrow, hypoplasia of, 48
Bones, 5
Bradycardia, 35
Bronchitis, acute, 38-39
  chronic, 38
  see also emphysema
Burns, 64, 124, 125

CALCIUM, 45, 117
Carbohydrate, 50, 118
Carbon dioxide, 35
Cardiac ouput, 33-34, 35
Cardiac reserve, 33
Cardio-vascular disease, 32-38
Catheter, nasal, for oxygen, 35
  urinary, 68, 113-115
Cerebral embolism, 27
Cerebral haemorrhage, 27
Cerebral thrombosis, 26
Cerebro-vascular accident,
  effects of, 27-29
  see also stroke
Cerebro-vascular disease, 26-32
Cervical spondylosis, 44
Chair, suitable for elderly patient, 142
  getting up from, 140
  sitting down in, 139
Chest diseases, 38-41
Chiropody, chiropodist, 151, 164
Circle of Willis, 26
Clinistix reagent, 49
Clubs, for the elderly, 166-167
  luncheon, 162
Compulsory admission, 20

Confidence, loss of, 58-60
Confusion, care of the patient
  with, 84-88
  at night, 89-90
  in the long-stay ward, 78
Confusional states (temporary
  acute toxic), 24, 53-54
Constipation, 69-70
  prevention of, 70
Contractures, 29, 42, 43
Coroner, 101
Cot-sides, 90-91
Coupling, 32, 35

DAY CARE, 165-167
Day centres, 166
Day hospital, 75-77
Day room, area, 74-75, 78
Deafness, 8, 91-93
  talking to the elderly deaf,
    91-92
Death, 12, 95-96
  certificate, 100
  grant, 101
  from pneumonia, 39-41
  registration of, 100
  see also dying
Degenerative conditions, 24
Delirious patients, 86-87
Dementia, 54-55
  care of the patient with, 84-87
  cerebro-arterio sclerotic, 54
  senile, 54
Dentist, 76
Dentures, 7
Department of Health and
  Social Security, 163
Depression, care of the patient
  with, 88
  endogenous, 56-57
  reactive, 55
Diabetes mellitus, 49-51
Diarrhoea, 69, 70
Diet, 116-120
  as a factor in constipation,
    69-70
  in diabetes, 50-51
Digitalis, digoxin, see drugs
Disabled Living Foundation,
  143
Discharge from hospital,
  153-158
  planned, 155-156

  extended, 156-158
Disengagement, 12
Diuretics, see drugs
Diversional activities,
  occupation, 78, 147-148
Domiciliary services, 158-165
  see also individual services
Drop attacks, 44
Dressing, 142
Drugs, accidental poisoning
  with, 64
  administration of, 122-123
  analgesics, 42, 43, 98
  antibiotics, 38-40, 63
  anti-depressants, 56, 88
  anti-diabetic, 50
  anti-Parkinsonism, 31
  anti-tubercular, 41
  aperients, 69
  barbiturates, 24
  digitalis, digoxin, 35-36
  diuretics, 36
  hypotensive, 36
  in iatrogenic disorders, 24
  iron, 46, 48
  sedatives, 90
  tranquillisers, 86
Dying, care of the, 95-99
Dysarthria, 28
Dysphasia, 28, 149

ECCHYMOSES, 5
Electro-convulsive therapy,
  56, 57
Endocrine disorders, 49-52
Enema, 70, 98
Euthanasia, 41
Exercises, assisted, 144
  for balance, 144
  end of bed, 137
  functional, 145
  group, 75
  passive, 129-130
  resisted, 144
Experimental day, weekend at
  home, 157
Extrinsic factor, 47

FAECES, IMPACTED, 69
Falls, 64-65, 124-125
Fasting blood sugar, 49
Feeding patients, 121
Fluid balance, 119-120

177

Fluids, 117
Foam pads, 107
Foot drop, 30
Foster homes, 171
Fractures, 44, 45, 63, 124

GANGRENE, 37, 50
Gas, 8, 64
General practitioner, 71, 159, 175
Geriatric care, future of, 173-174
  history of, 1, 172
  improvements in, 173
  nature of, 72, 172
Gerontology, 1
Glucose tolerance test, 7, 49
Good Neighbour scheme, 22, 165
Grand-parent, rôle of, 11-12

HAEMOGLOBIN, 45-48
Half-way house, 77, 157-158
Health education, 6, 174-175
Health visitor, 160-161, 163, 173
Hearing aids, 92
Heart, 6
Heart disease, ischaemic, 34
  pulmonary, 34
  valvular, 34
Heart failure, 33-36
Heat treatment, 42, 44, 146
Heating, domestic, 21, 61-63
Hemiparesis, 27
Hemiplegia, 27
Histamine test meal, 47
Holiday support for relatives, 58
Holidays, 164
Home help, 161-162
Home nurse, 159-160
Home visit, by geriatrician, 71-73
Homes, Old People's, 19, 169-171
  day care in, 167
  charitable, 170
  local authority, 169-170
  private, 170-171
Homonymous hemianopia, 29
Hospital Advisory Service, 172-173
Hospital chaplain, 96, 151
Hydrochloric acid, 46, 47-48

Hypertension, 36-37
Hyperthyroidism, *see* thyrotoxicosis
Hypoglycaemia, 50
Hypotension, 48
Hypothermia, 25, 60-63
  prevention of, 60
  treatment of, 62
Hypothyroidism, *see* myxoedema

IATROGENIC DISORDERS, 24
Incomes, 16-17
Incontinence, of faeces, 69
  of urine, accidental, 65-67
  in long-stay wards, 78
  management of, 110-115
  nocturnal, 66
  pathological, 66-69
Insulin, 49
Intelligence, 9-10
Intermittent claudication, 37
Intrinsic factor, 46-48
Involution, 4
Iron, 45-46, 117, *see also* drugs

JOINTS AFFECTED IN ARTHRITIS, 41-44

KIDNEYS, 6

LAUNDRY SERVICE, 163
Leisure, 11, 12
Library service, 164
Lifting, 125-126
  Australian Lift, 126
Lip reading, 8, 92
Local authority, services provided by, 161-163
Loneliness, 19-20
Long-stay ward, 77-80
  nursing care in, 78-79
  patients in, 79-80
  poor conditions in, 172
Lungs, 6

MALIGNANT DISEASE, 24
Malnutrition, 117
Meals-on-wheels, 162
Memory, 10
Ménière's disease, 65
Mental testing, 88-89
Mouth care, 115-116

Moving house, home, 17, 167
Multiple pathology, 23
Muscle, 5
Music therapy, 149
Myxoedema, 51

NASO-GASTRIC TUBE, feeding by, 121-122
National Assistance Act, 1948 (Part 3), 91, 169
Neuritis, in diabetes, 50
  peripheral, 47
Night sitter service, 160

OBESITY, 118
Occupational therapy, 147-149
  community occupational therapist, 163
  in long-stay ward, 79
Old people's welfare committees, 22, 164
Optician, 7
Osteophytes, 42, 44
Osteoporosis, 44-45
Otosclerosis, 8
Outpatient clinic, department, 71, 73
Oxygen, administration of, 35, 41, 99

PACEMAKER, 33
Pain, 9, 25, 98
Palpitations, 32
Paraphrenia (late), 57
Paraplegia in anaemia, 47
Paresis, 27
Parkinson's disease, 30-32
Paroxysmal tachycardia, 32
Pensions, 16-17
Peripheral vascular disease, 37
Physiotherapy, physiotherapist, 30, 31, 39
  in rehabilitation, 143-146
Pneumonia, 39-41, 63
Population changes, 15
Post-mortem examination, 101
Postural drainage, 39
Posture, 5
Potassium, 36
Presbyopia, 7
Pressure sores, 102-109
  deep sores, 103
  prevention of, 105-108
  superficial sores, 103
  treatment, 105-109
Primary care team, 158-159, 174
Privacy, 84, 85
Progressive care, 71, 172
Prostate gland, 68
Pseudobulbar palsy, 27, 121
Psychogeriatric assessment ward, 80
Psychogeriatric day hospital, 76
Public transport, 18, 21
Pulse, 25
  dysrhythmias, 32

RE-ABLEMENT, 1, 129
Rectal dyschezia, 70
Reflexes, 6
Rehabilitation, 129-152
  assessment of capability and need, 130-131
  patient's attitude to, 132
  programmes, 134
  relatives' attitude to, 133-134
  rôle of doctor, 134-135
  rôle of nurse, 135-143
  ward, 74-75
Relatives, attitude to discharge, 155
  attitude to rehabilitation, 133-134
  involved in rehabilitation, 150
  patient moving to live with, 167-168
  of dying patient, 99-100
Religion, religious convictions, 12, 96
Renal failure, 98
  threshold for sugar, 6, 49
Respiration rate, 25
Restraining patient, 86-87, 91
Retinopathy, 36
  diabetic, 50
Retirement, 9-10
Ring pessary, 67
Ripple bed, 43, 106
Rotation system, 58
Roughage, 69, 117

SALT, 36
Seaside resorts, 15, 18
Senescence, 4, 6
Serving food, 120-121

Sheltered accommodation, housing, 19, 168-169
Shock, in accidents, 63, 124
 in hypothermia, 61
Shoes, 143
Sight, 7, 93-94
Skeletal system, diseases of, 41-45
Skin, 5
 applications to pressure areas, 107
 in hypothermia, 62
Sleep, 89-91
Sphincter, anal, 69
 bladder, 65-66
Splints, 145
Stokes Adams attacks, 33
Stress, 24
 incontinence, 67-69
Strokes, in long-stay ward, 79-80
 nursing care in, 29-30
 rehabilitation after, 134, 150
 see also cerebro-vascular accident
Sub-acute combined degeneration of the spinal cord, 47
Suicide, 56

TASTE, 7
Teeth, care of, 115
Telephone, 164
Temperature, 25
 in hypothermia, 60-63
Thermometer, low reading, 25

Thirst, 97
Thyrotoxicosis, 51-52
Transient ischaemic attacks, 26
Tremor, in Parkinson's disease, 31
 in thyrotoxicosis, 52
Tuberculosis, pulmonary, 41
Turning the patient, 127-128

URINE, 6, 65-69, 110-112
 infection of, 68
 retention with overflow, 67-68
 specific gravity of, 6
Ultra-violet light treatment, 109, 146

VERTEBRAE, 5, 44, 45
Vitamin B_{12}, 46-48
Vitamin C, 117
Voluntary helpers in hospital, 79, 151
Voluntary visitor, 20, 164
Vomiting, in the dying, 99

WALKING, 138, 145
 with frame 138-140, 146
Warts, senile, 5
Water mattress, 106
Wheelchair, 37, 145
Wills, 100
Wrist drop, 29
W.R.V.S., 162

X-RAY DEPARTMENT, 73

ZIMMER FRAME, 138-139, 145

Other books in the Nursing Modules Series...

PSYCHIATRIC CARE & CONDITIONS introduces the student nurse to the basic facts, concepts and principles of modern psychiatric nursing and will give her a reasonable insight into the problems of the psychiatric patient, the treatment he will receive and the people involved in his care.

0 85602 029 X   160 pages

OBSTETRIC CARE is about childbirth and the people involved. It provides the student nurse with the essential information necessary to her course and by accentuating the principles and approach to good nursing practice, will help her to develop skill and confidence.

0 85602 027 3   192 pages

COMMUNITY CARE examines the health and social services and the work of the community health team. It describes how the sick and other vulnerable groups are cared for in the community setting, and will help the student to understand the very different pattern of nursing involved.

0 85602 028 1   160 pages